CW01497815

THE
MARY
STANFORD
DISASTER

THE STORY OF A LIFEBOAT
NOVEMBER 15, 1928

GEOFF HUTCHINSON

DEDICATED TO
THE MEMORY OF
THE CREW OF
THE MARY STANFORD LIFEBOAT
1928

It was not among the battle's din,
Nor goaded on to slay;
But to save the lives of strangers,
They met their deaths this day

Mrs E J Veness, 1928

First published 1984
Revised edition 1993

ISBN 0 9519936 1 5

Design, artwork and typesetting by the author
Text set in 10/12pt Century Book
Printed by M & W Morgan, Red Lake Terrace, Ore, Hastings

Contents

Foreword

The Rye Harbour lifeboat disaster, in which *The Mary Stanford* was capsized and 17 men lost their lives, was doubly tragic as the sailors they set out to rescue had already been saved before the lifeboat launched. This message reached the lifeboat house too late and recall signals were not seen by the lifeboatmen. They searched in vain and were on their way home when tragedy struck.

With modern communications, such a disaster would have been avoided as the lifeboat would not have been launched. However, lifeboatmen today are still prepared to face the gruelling storms which the Rye Harbour crew faced over half a century ago. They know that even with the finest boats and equipment, there is a risk and yet they set out to help complete strangers.

The book records a grim episode in the RNLI's history and reminds us of the tremendous sacrifices over the years by our lifeboatmen. The Rye Harbour memorial speaks for all RNLI crews 'We have done that which was our duty to do'.

Rear Admiral W J Graham CB MNI
The Director, RNLI, 1979-87

Other titles by the same author:

FULLER OF SUSSEX — A Georgian Squire

GREY OWL — The incredible story of Archie Belaney, 1888-1938

BAIRD — The story of John Logie Baird, 1888-1946

HUMGRUFFIN — A story of country folk . . . and giants

THE LOVERS' SEAT — The history and the love story of 1786. Fact and fiction

KIPLING — Rudyard Kipling, 1865-1936. An introduction

AN INTRODUCTION TO HASTINGS & ST LEONARDS

AN INTRODUCTION TO BEXHILL-ON-SEA

AN INTRODUCTION TO BATTLE, RYE AND THE VILLAGES

Introduction

The month of November is a time of remembrance. At numerous ceremonies across the land the fallen of the great wars are honoured for their bravery and personal sacrifice. It is a time of mixed emotions; of sadness and thoughts of what might have been, but mostly it is a time of enduring pride.

For the inhabitants of the tiny fishing village of Rye Harbour in East Sussex there is an added poignancy. For each year on the Sunday closest to November 15, the parish church at Rye Harbour is always full. The unique remembrance service which takes place recalls a day nearly 70 years ago, when the community was devastated, not by an act of war, but as the result of an appalling disaster.

Rye Harbour is situated in Rye Bay between Hastings and Dungeness and has approximately 400 inhabitants. In the late 1920s the population was even smaller and the majority of the close-knit community gained its livelihood from the sea and where men put to sea in ships there is usually a lifeboat.

The Mary Stanford was the fifth lifeboat to serve the dangerous waters of Rye Bay. This is the true story of that lifeboat and the courage of its crew, a story of the sea and the cruel irony played on the willing men of that boat. In the true tradition of the lifeboat service the crew answered the call of duty in treacherous weather conditions — the worst in living memory — to be sent on, as it turned out, a pointless mission, resulting in one of the worst disasters ever known in the lifeboat service.

Through the ages there have been many tales of heroism connected to the sea, but surely few can match the selfless courage and sacrifice of the men of the Rye Harbour lifeboat who were called to duty on a fateful November day in 1928.

This is an account of the happenings of that day, its aftermath, and the bravery of the crew of *The Mary Stanford.*

LIST OF SERVICES RENDERED BY THE
RYE HARBOUR LIFEBOATS
OF THE
ROYAL NATIONAL LIFE-BOAT INSTITUTION, 1852-1928.

LIVES RESCUED FROM SHIPWRECK

FIRST LIFEBOAT.

1852	August 15	Brig, "Avon," of London	::	::	3
1862	December 10	American Ship, "James Browne"	::	::	18
1867	January 23	Barque, "Marie Amelie," of Quimper.	Assisted to save Vessel and		14
	February 1	Brigantine, "Estelle," of Preston.	Saved Vessel	::	

SECOND LIFEBOAT.
The "STORM SPRITE," gift of the Solicitors' and Proctors' Lifeboat Fund.

1867	October 22	Ship, "Michiels Loos," of Antwerp.	Stood by Vessel	::	
1869	February 14	Brig, "Pearl," of Shoreham	::	::	8
1871	January 16	Brig, "Elizabeth & Cicely," of Guernsey	::	::	8
	December 18	Barque, "Robina," of North Shields	::	::	8
1874	February 25	Schooner, "Helene," of Cranz	::	::	4
1876	January 21	Brig, "Fred Thompson," of Dundee.	Stood by Vessel		
1877	December 22	Schooner, "Vier Broders," of Groningen	::	::	4
1878	January 28	Schooner, "Fearless," of Guernsey	::	::	6

THIRD LIFEBOAT.
The "FRANCES HARRIS," legacy of the late Mrs. Harris, of Streatham.

1884	January 23	Brig, "Silksworth," of Blyth	::	::	7
1890	December 4	Steam Tug, No. 15, of Plymouth.	Assisted to save Vessel and		6
1891	December 28	Barque, "Warwickshire," of London	::	::	18
1896	December 5	S.S. "Menzaleh," of London.	Rendered assistance	::	

FOURTH LIFEBOAT.
The "JOHN WILLIAM DUDLEY," legacy of the late Mr. J. W. Dudley, of Woodford.

1900	October 25	Ship, "Helicon," of Hamburg.	Rendered assistance	::	
1901	January 19	Cutter, "Jeune Arthur," of Cherbourg	::	::	4
1902	February 23	Ketch, "Pilot," of Plymouth.	Saved Vessel and	::	4
1904	Feb. 20-25	S.S. "Lake Michigan," of Liverpool.	Stood by Vessel	::	
	May 2	Ship, "Derwent," of London.	Stood by Vessel	::	
1905	June 22	S.S. "Clara," of London.	Stood by Vessel	::	
1907	January 22	Ketch, "Lord Tennyson," of London.	Rescued 3 and a dog	::	3
	March 18	S.S. "Swan," of Sunderland.	Stood by Vessel		
1909	December 22	S.S. "Salatis," of Hamburg.	Rendered assistance	::	
	December 22	Boat of Tug, "Oceana," of London.	::	::	3
1910	March 9	Steam Trawler, "Margaret," of Rye.	Stood by Vessel	::	
1912	December 26	S.S. "Bedeburn," of Newcastle.	Assisted to save Vessel	::	
1916	April 17	S.S. "Kirnwood," of Middlesborough.	Rendered assistance	::	

FIFTH LIFEBOAT.
The "MARY STANFORD," legacy of the late Mr. John Stanford.

1920	May 28	S.S. "Thora Fredrikke," of Porsgrund.	Stood by Vessel		
1921	March 29	Barge, "Lady Ellen," of Woodbridge.	::		2
1923	February 27	Motor Schooner, "Alice," of Falmouth	::		8
	December 13	Aeroplane G.E.B.T. (Sperry)	Helped Aeroplane	

The boat . . .

In May 1914, a decision was made by the Royal National Lifeboat Institution to offer the Rye Harbour station a new lifeboat. The existing vessel, the self-righting *John William Dudley*, which had been in operation since 1900, was reaching the end of a distinguished working career, during which time she had been launched 42 times, saving 14 lives. The Institution considered it time to ring the changes.

The coxswain, Herbert Head and two other crew members were invited to visit other lifeboat stations to see the types of boat available and, during the following months, travelled the length and breadth of the country, inspecting several different kinds of vessel, working under the same conditions as those experienced at Rye Harbour. As a result, they eventually chose a Liverpool-type class, a surf-boat specially constructed for the type of flat coastline to be found in the Rye area. These boats, although not able to self-right, were larger and more stable and were able to go well out to sea. They were also easier to launch. Self-righting boats such as *The John William Dudley* were heavier and drew more water and caused added problems in getting away from the shore. Due to the flatness of its surroundings and the long tides experienced in the area, it was impractical to construct a slipway at the Rye Harbour station, meaning that the lifeboat had to be manhandled across the beach into the water. Therefore, a lighter vessel, which would minimise the effort of launching, was considered a most welcome and suitable replacement. Nine Liverpool-type boats were in use around this time and during the 10 years they were in service 1,120 lives were saved.

However, as it was not a self-righting boat, there were mixed feelings about the choice of this type of vessel among the community at Rye Harbour. The local assistant honorary secretary of the RNLI expressed grave doubts about its suitability, but it was the crew who had the final say. They were always consulted about the type of craft they would prefer and no boat was ever given to a crew unless they expressed complete satisfaction.

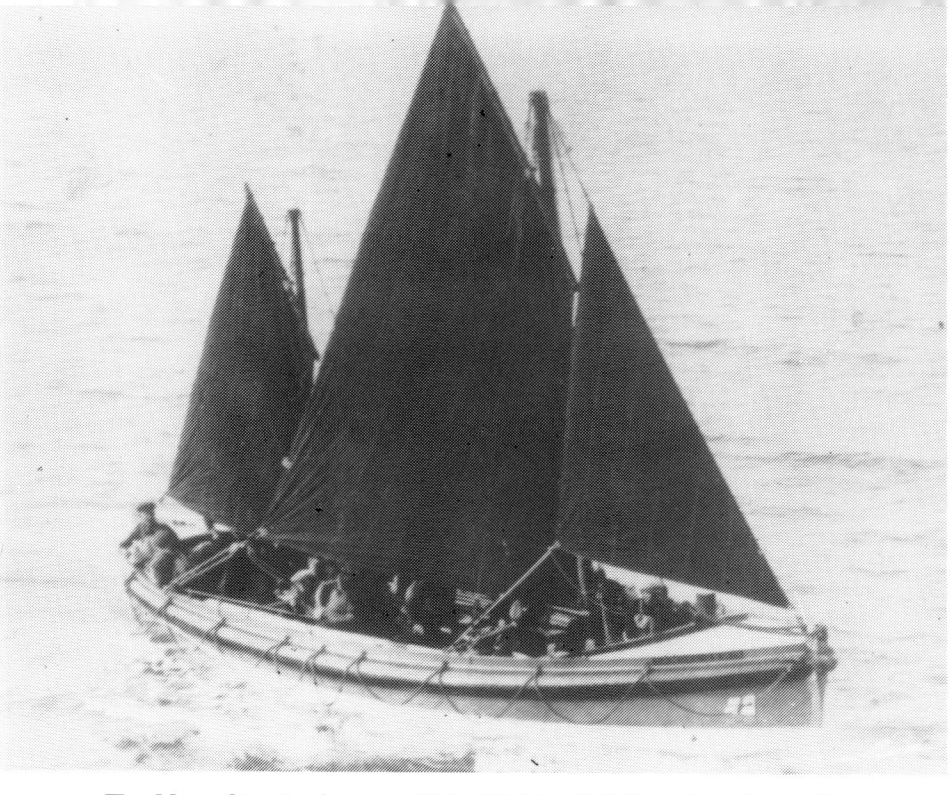

The Mary Stanford was built in 1916 by S E Saunders Ltd at East Cowes, on the Isle of Wight, at a cost of £2,173. She was 38ft long by 10ft 9in wide, and her weight complete was 4 tons 12¼ cwts. Lifeboats in those days were crude by today's standards. They had no engine and carried no radio. The Liverpool-type class was a pulling and sailing vessel, propelled by oars and a close-reefed mainsail. An extremely high level of seamanship and dedication was necessary to sail such a vessel and the physical demands placed on its crew were enormous. It was certainly not a job for the faint-hearted.

The Mary Stanford was purchased from the continuing legacy of a Mr John Stanford of Regents Park, London, a great admirer of the lifeboat service, who had earlier bequeathed a large sum of money to have a lifeboat built and dedicated to the memory of his mother. It was the second boat serving the south coast to carry her name. The first *Mary Stanford* was given in 1881 to the Rye Lifeboat station, which operated from a boathouse situated on Camber Sands. This Rye station was later closed and its duties taken over by Rye Harbour station in 1910.

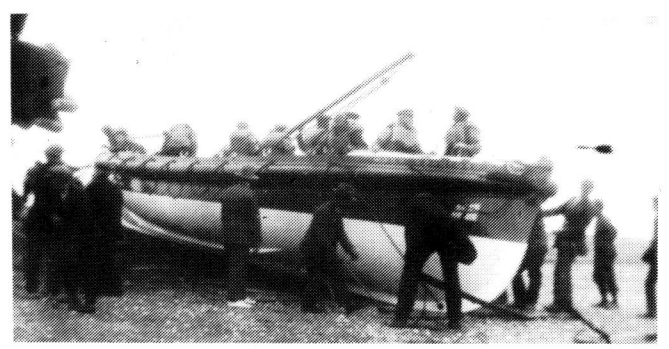

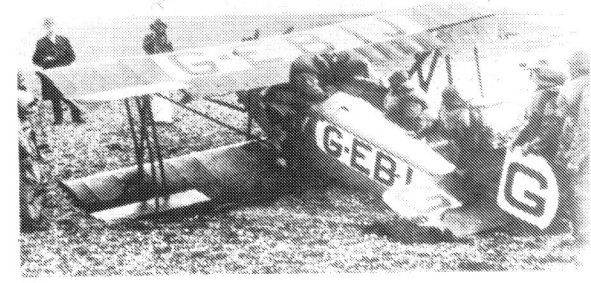

Above: A practice launch.
Right: The aircraft, Sperry
Messenger, towed ashore by
The Mary Stanford in
December 1923

Facing page: A Liverpool-
type class lifeboat

So the second *Mary Stanford*, after being thoroughly tested for draft and stability by the makers on April 13, 1916, was eventually sailed from East Cowes to Rye Harbour by the crew and placed on service at the station on October 19, 1916. On November 25 of that year a test exercise was carried out at Rye under weather conditions that gave the boat a stern test of its capabilities and she passed with flying colours. The crew had complete faith in their new lifeboat.

During her time at Rye Harbour *The Mary Stanford* was launched on 63 occasions, 47 times in practise and 16 times on active service. Perhaps the most spectacular of her missions was in December 1923, when she was launched to attend an aircraft which had ditched in the sea near Fairlight. The pilot, an American, L B Sperry, had been flying from Croydon bound for Amsterdam. Although the lifeboat was able to tow the plane to shore, the pilot had attempted to swim for shore and was lost.

However, there were many successes and during 12 years' service at Rye Harbour, *The Mary Stanford* and her crew were responsible for saving 10 lives from the waters of Rye Bay.

... The crew

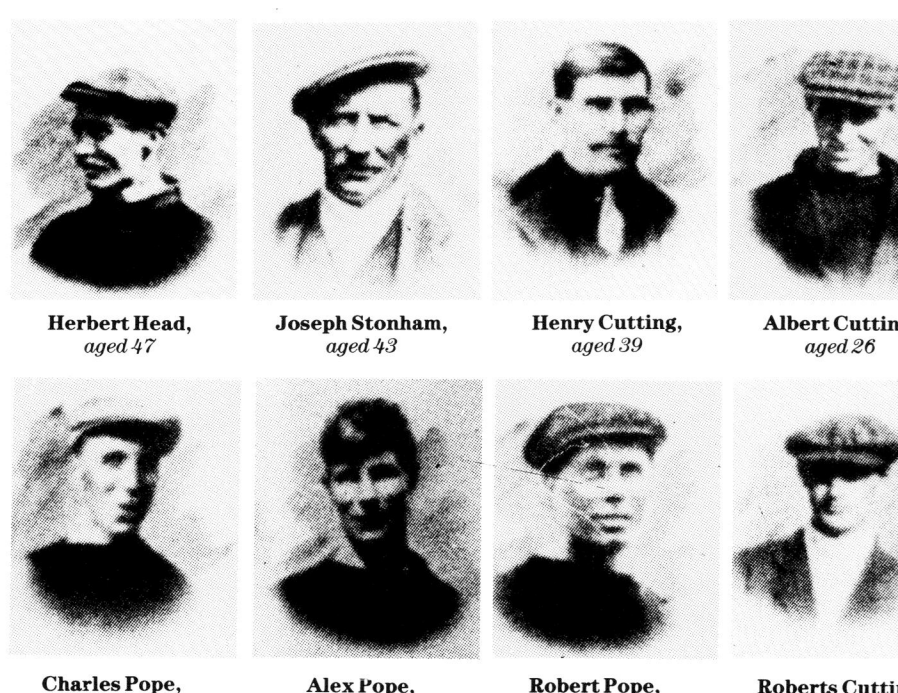

Herbert Head,
aged 47

Joseph Stonham,
aged 43

Henry Cutting,
aged 39

Albert Cutting,
aged 26

Charles Pope,
aged 28

Alex Pope,
aged 21

Robert Pope,
aged 23

Roberts Cutting,
aged 28

Since the lifeboat service began in 1824, its boats have always been manned by volunteers; men who, in addition to their everyday jobs, have always been prepared to sacrifice their leisure time and comfort and put their own lives at risk for the safety of others.

The crew of the Rye Harbour lifeboat in 1928 were drawn from the young men of the village. The average age was 29 years. Many were fishermen and all were experienced seamen; friends who had grown up together and worked with each other in the tiny close-knit community. A number of them were married and many were related.

The coxswain was Mr Herbert Head, a married man, aged 47 years, whose two sons were also in the crew. Joseph Stonham (43) was second coxswain, and Henry Cutting, aged 39, was the bowman.

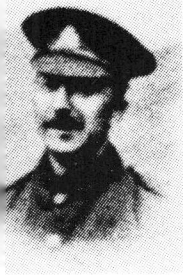

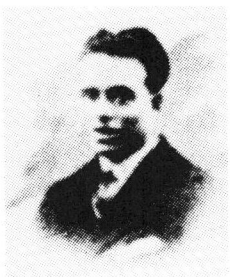

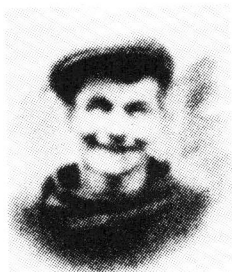

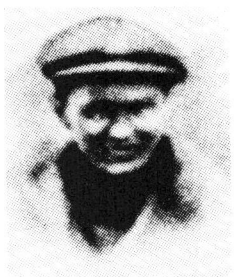

Walter Igglesden,
aged 38

Charles Southerden,
aged 22

James Head,
aged 19

John Head,
aged 17

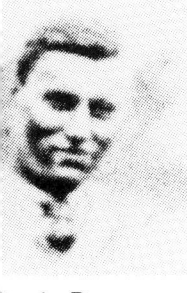

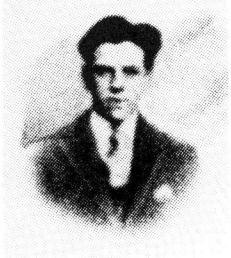

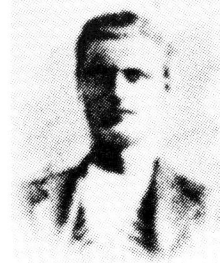

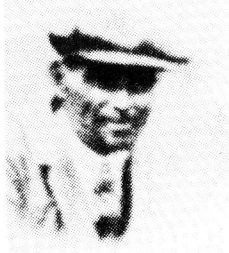

Morriss Downey,
aged 23

Arthur Downey,
aged 25

Leslie Clark,
aged 24

William Clark,
aged 27

The men of the

Mary Stanford lifeboat

November 15, 1928

Albert Smith,
aged 44

The storm

The month of November can bring terrible storms to the waters of Rye Bay and the weather conditions during the evening of Wednesday November 14, 1928 and into the following day, were some of the worst ever experienced. South-westerly gales up to 80mph, accompanied by driving rain, swept across the area, whipping the sea into huge waves. Someone remarked at the time: 'I don't think I've seen as much sea in Rye Bay as there was that day.' The spray was driven over four miles inland by the incessant wind blowing off the shallow breaking water. It hung over the village of Rye Harbour like a thick mist. Visibility was down to a few yards and the salt mist browned the trees on the weather side.

As the people of Rye Harbour retired to their beds that night, they prayed the lifeboat would not have to be launched, but in their hearts they knew it was more than a distinct possibility.

As the night drew on and the storm worsened, many ships in the English Channel found themselves in increasing difficulties. Most successfully made for shelter in Folkestone or Dover, but some were not so fortunate. At around 4am an incident took place which set off a chain of events which would end in bitter tragedy for the people of Rye Harbour.

The Latvian ship, *The Alice of Riga* laden with bricks, was struggling through the heavy seas, south-west of Dungeness, when she became involved in a collision with the larger German steamer, *The Smyrna. The Alice*, her rudder gone and a hole torn in her side, began taking in water and drifting helplessly in the heavy seas and violent storm.

The captain of *The Smyrna* kept his vessel close by, but the darkness and severity of the weather stopped him being able to offer any practical assistance to the crew of the stricken *Alice*. He decided he would have to wait until daybreak before any rescue attempt could be mounted. In the meantime he sent out the following message, which was received by the North Foreland radio station and passed on to the Liaison Officer at Ramsgate Coastguard Station. It read: *Steamer Alice Riga leaking — danger — drifting SW to W 8 miles from Dungeness 0430.*

The Rye Harbour Coastguard Station was informed at 4.50am and the lifeboat was soon to be alerted.

The die was cast. The fate of the men of *The Mary Stanford* was sealed.

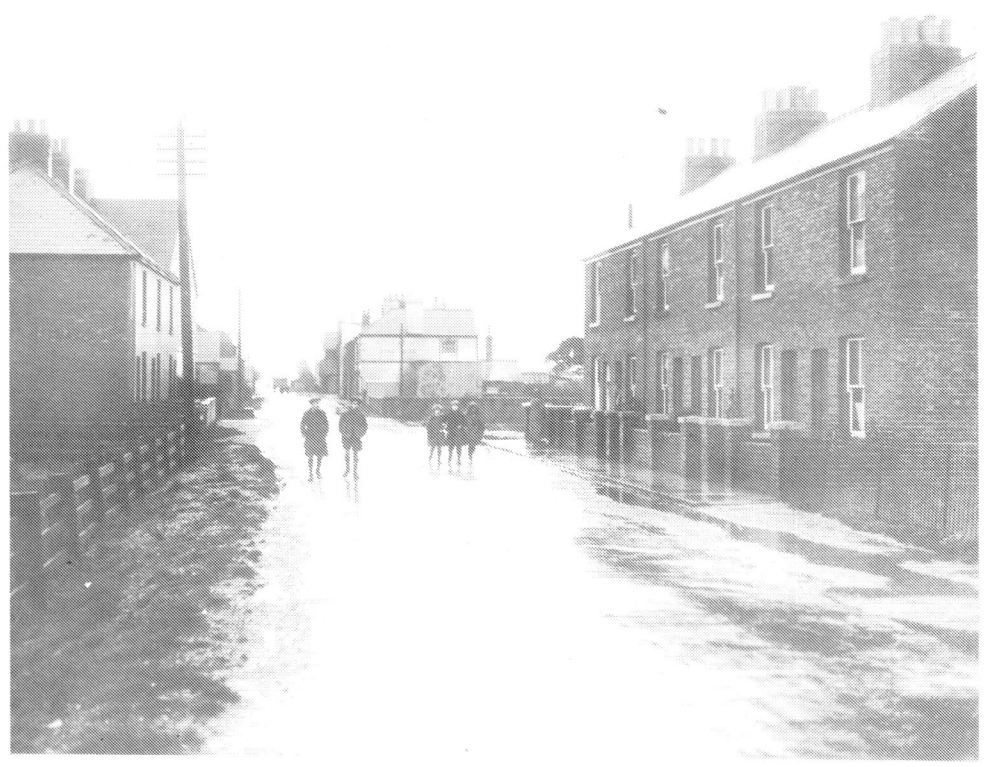

Rye Harbour, circa 1928

November 15, 1928

It was just after 5am when the maroon called the crew of *The Mary Stanford* to duty.

Swiftly the crew tumbled from their beds, donned their gear and raced out into the streets. The vicar of Rye Harbour, the Rev Harry Newton, remarking on the speed of their response, declared that 'it was as if they had slept with their clothes on'.

Rushed and sometimes heated conversations ensued in some households as members of the families determined just exactly who would man the lifeboat in such severe weather. Younger members persuaded older members not to go, and took their places. Walter Igglesden was at first refused permission to go by his father, but managed to persuade him otherwise. It was to be Lewis Pope's first trip on active service and his heart must have been thumping fast as he sped out of the house with two of his more experienced brothers, Robert and Charles.

One crewman had spent the past weeks and days planning his forthcoming wedding, but now there were other things to think of as he rushed off into the wind-swept night.

One young member of the crew, Arthur Robus, had been working late the previous night and his mother tried anxiously to rouse him from his deep sleep. She failed and he missed the launch. Major W B Hacking, a committee member of the RNLI at Rye Harbour, was another to miss the launch. He lived on the outskirts of Rye near the village of Udimore, and it was his practice, on hearing the maroon, to leap on a horse and charge across the fields and shingle to the lifeboat house. But this morning the sound of the maroon could not be heard above the roaring of the wind.

Herbert Head, the coxswain reassured his wife about the safety of himself and his two sons before rushing away. Such were the bustling scenes that morning as the men sped off to do their duty. On a morning when most people would not even put their noses out the door, the men of the Rye Harbour lifeboat did not know the meaning of the word 'hesitation'. There were lives to be saved. As Mrs Head remarked: 'They just went!'

It was not just the crew that jumped into action. Sometimes up to 60 launchers were involved in getting the boat off. Nobody was turned away, lives were at risk. 'Get the boat off! Get the boat off!' was the cry — whatever the weather.

The lifeboat house at Rye Harbour was about a mile and a half from the village and the crew and launchers had an exhausting dash, their bodies bent double into the gale force wind, across rough shingle, fields, fences and obstacles of all kinds . . . in the pitch dark. By the time they reached the boathouse they were already drenched to the skin.

The tide that morning was at its lowest point, which meant it would be a difficult launch, because as the tide begins to rise again the weather gets worse. There was no tractor to pull *The Mary Stanford* into the sea and she had to be dragged by brute force over a

The boathouse still stands today on the lonely stretch of beach between Rye Harbour and Winchelsea Beach

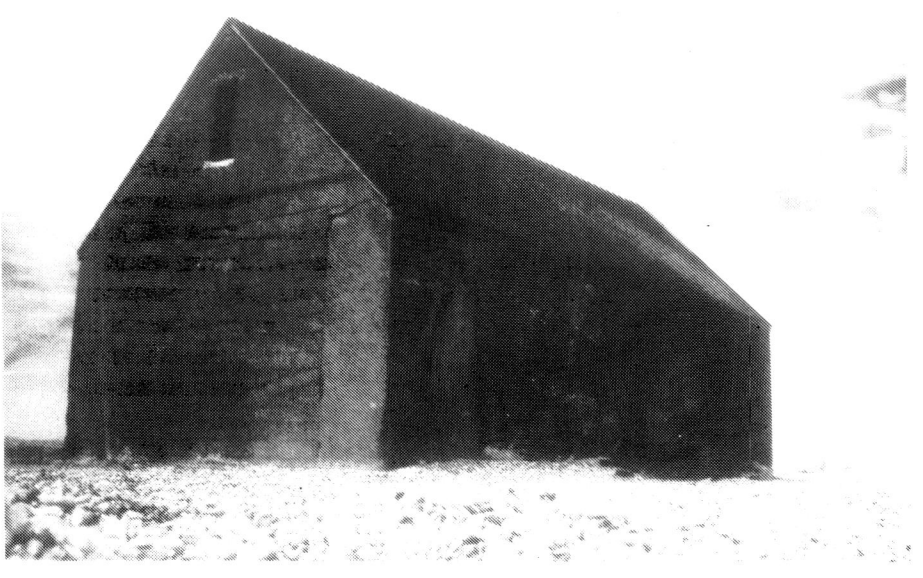

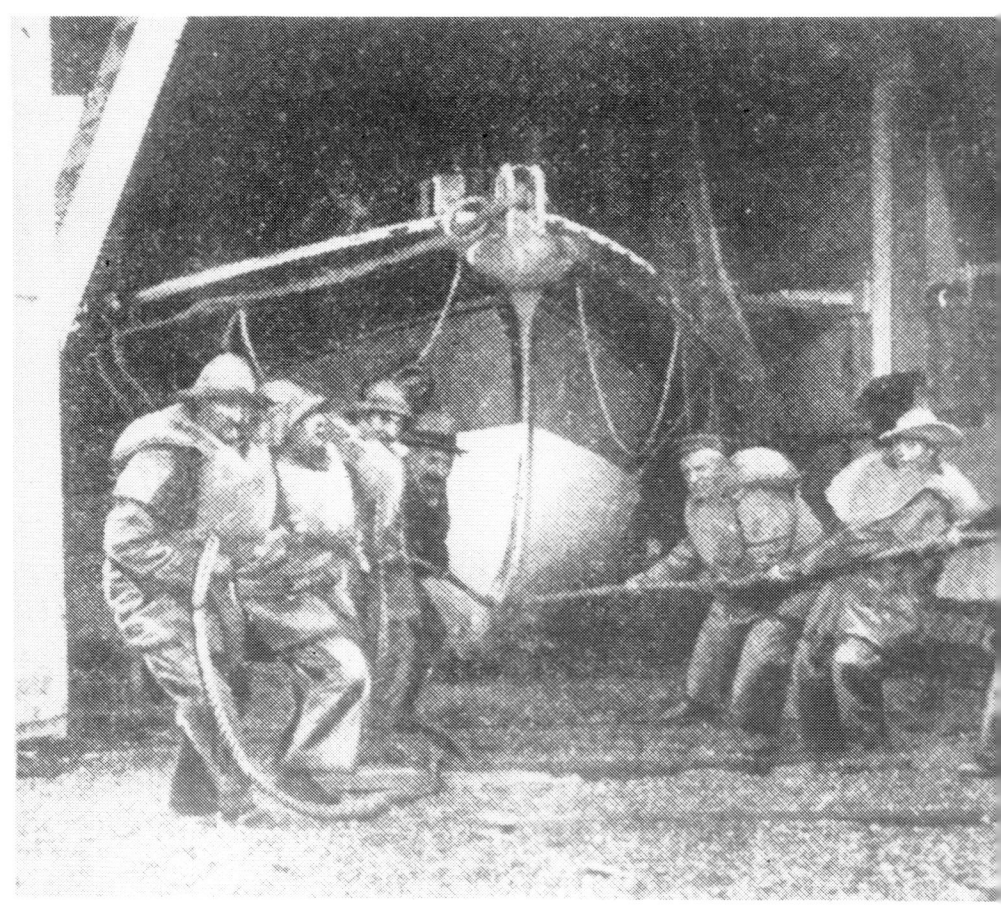

distance of approximately 1000 yards across beach and sand to the sea. Heavily greased skids were placed across the beach and a rope wreathed through the bow of the boat and with launchers either side, the craft was pulled painstakingly towards the sea. They had to wade into the water until there was enough depth for the boat to float and the foremost of these men had to be immersed to their shoulders.

On the first attempt to get her away *The Mary Stanford* was blown back on to the shore. Another try was made and the same thing happened. The weather was worsening by the minute as the launchers struggled in the most dangerous circumstances to get the boat away from the beach. They faced the increasing risk of being crushed under the heaving vessel as it crashed back onto the shore.

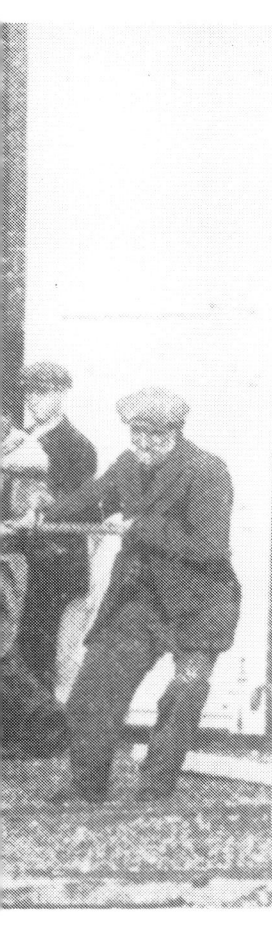

The Mary Stanford had to be hauled from the boathouse across the beach to the sea

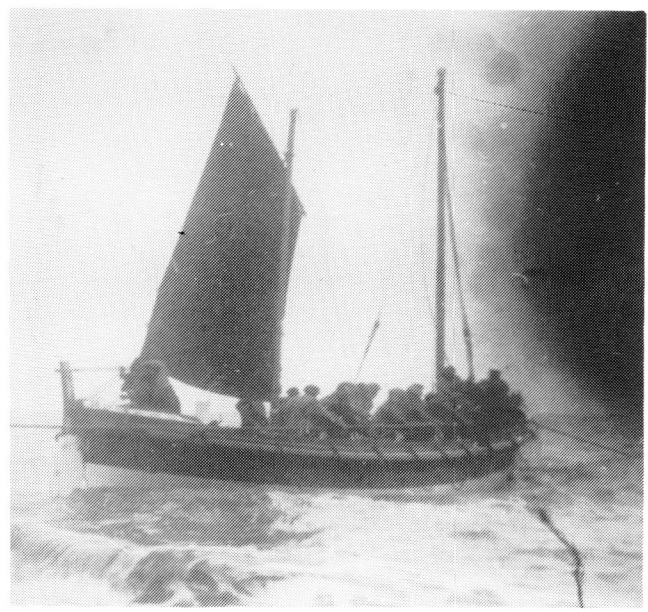

At last, on the third attempt, at approximately 6.45am, *The Mary Stanford* finally got away. The crew now had to face the daunting task of setting the boat's sail and rowing through the high, rough, broken sea. It is said that even before they were afloat the 17 men of the crew were exhausted after that launch.

The next sad twist to the story came as a message was received by the Rye coastguards at 6.50am stating that the crew of the stricken *Alice* had been rescued by the *Smyrna,* and the lifeboat's assistance was no longer required. The message was transmitted immediately to the lifeboat house. It had been received from the North Foreland radio station by Ramsgate Coastguard Station at 6.12am.

The question of how long this message took to arrive at the lifeboat house was to cause much debate. The regulations which existed at that time stated that priority be given over other telegraphic and telephonic messages to those calling for the services of a lifeboat. However, there was no such priority given to a message which stated that the services were *not* required and it is highly probable that any delay was due to this ruling.

Hence *The Mary Stanford* had been afloat about five minutes when the message was received. There was no ship to shore radio in those days and the boat had to be recalled by flares.

Frantically the signalman fired the recall signal and men raced into the water with loud-hailers to stop the lifeboat. But by now the crew must have been too occupied in getting the sails set and did not acknowledge the signal. Two more white Verey lights — the recognised recall for a lifeboat — were fired; all to no avail. Facing out to sea, with a 15ft oar in their hands and sails to set in a gale of wind, and with spray and teeming rain blowing into them, it is small wonder they never saw the all-important recall signal.

And so the 17 men of the lifeboat spent several hours in Rye Bay on a pointless mission in weather conditions which worsened as daylight came.

At around 9am, the lifeboat was seen by the mate of the *SS Halton*, WSW 3 miles from Dungeness as she passed at a distance of about half a mile, with two small tug sails set. He stated that all was well with her.

It was at the entrance of Rye Harbour as she eventually made for home that *The Mary Stanford* capsized at about 10.30am when she was 1½ miles from safety. This made it a double tragedy. Not only had she gone on a wasted journey, she was so near to home when she was engulfed by a giant wave and overturned. It happened on the harbour bar, an area of shallow water where long waves that roll up the Channel, break as they hit the sandbanks, and become steep and irregular. As she crashed over on her side, her mast snapped and the crew were thrown into the heavy seas.

The harbour master at the time later expressed surprise that the crew had even attempted to return to Rye Harbour at all. On previous occasions, when gales were less fierce, the boat had gone on to Folkestone, not returning until the weather had subsided.

But not this time . . .

Later that day

By mid-morning the rumours began to filter through. The most widely-accepted reasoning for the boat not returning was that she had sought shelter in the lee of Dungeness or Folkestone Harbour as the men waited for the storm to subside before returning home. Stories of capsize were quickly dismissed. In the minds of the people of Rye Harbour, that just could not happen.

The villagers had great faith in their lifeboat and menfolk and, although they were naturally worried for their safety, there were no dark thoughts in their minds. There was certainly no talk of tragedy. The lifeboatmen had just gone to do a job of work; they would be back sooner or later.

Everyone knew the men were all experienced seamen and had often gone out fishing for long periods, sometimes for several days at a time and many times in bad weather. They were confident the men knew how to look after themselves and the people of Rye Harbour set about their daily business as usual. Sadly this day would have a far from happy ending.

Between 10 and 11 o'clock that morning a youngster named Cecil Marchant, of Camber, was walking along the sands collecting driftwood. The tide was about three parts in when he saw a boat returning to harbour in very rough seas. He saw the mast of the boat going over as the craft disappeared under a huge wave. He knew the lifeboat had been launched as he had heard the maroon fired earlier and he raced home to inform his parents. They disbelieved him. Mr and Mrs Marchant, along with many others, were of the misguided opinion that lifeboats just could not capsize. However, the boy's father quickly informed the coastguard station at Jurys Gap and at around 12 o'clock the worst fears were confirmed as the lifeboat was seen, bottom upwards, floating towards the shore.

Within 10 minutes the Rye coastguard station was informed. A maroon was fired, which people in Rye Harbour thought was a signal to the launchers to bring the boat in. The vicar, who had also witnessed the boat capsize, as he looked out from the vicarage windows, was quickly out on the street to tell the assembled launchers the bad news. There was an air of disbelief that such a thing could have happened.

Everything that was humanly possible was done. The Hastings lifeboat was summoned but could not be launched as the sea was too rough. A hundred men, including the rocket crew, coastguards carrying lifebelts, policemen and willing helpers were rushed to the beach, where the upturned boat now lay. Frantic attempts were made to right the boat, but as the craft weighed over four tons, they proved unsuccessful. A tank from the nearby army camp at Lydd was immediately sent for and it carefully pulled the boat on to its side. Two men were found trapped beneath, wedged between the seats of the boat. Walter Igglesden was alive, his body still warm, but extensive attempts to revive him failed.

Soon the full horror of the disaster became apparent as one by one the bodies of the lifeboatmen were washed, battered and bruised, towards the shore. Artificial respiration was administered but it was

A tank from the nearby Lydd army camp was used to pull the boat on to its side

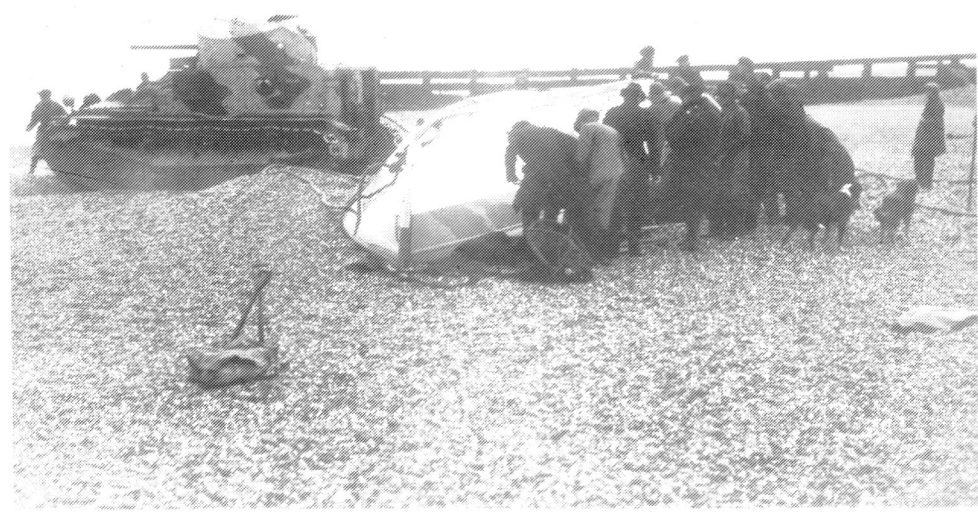

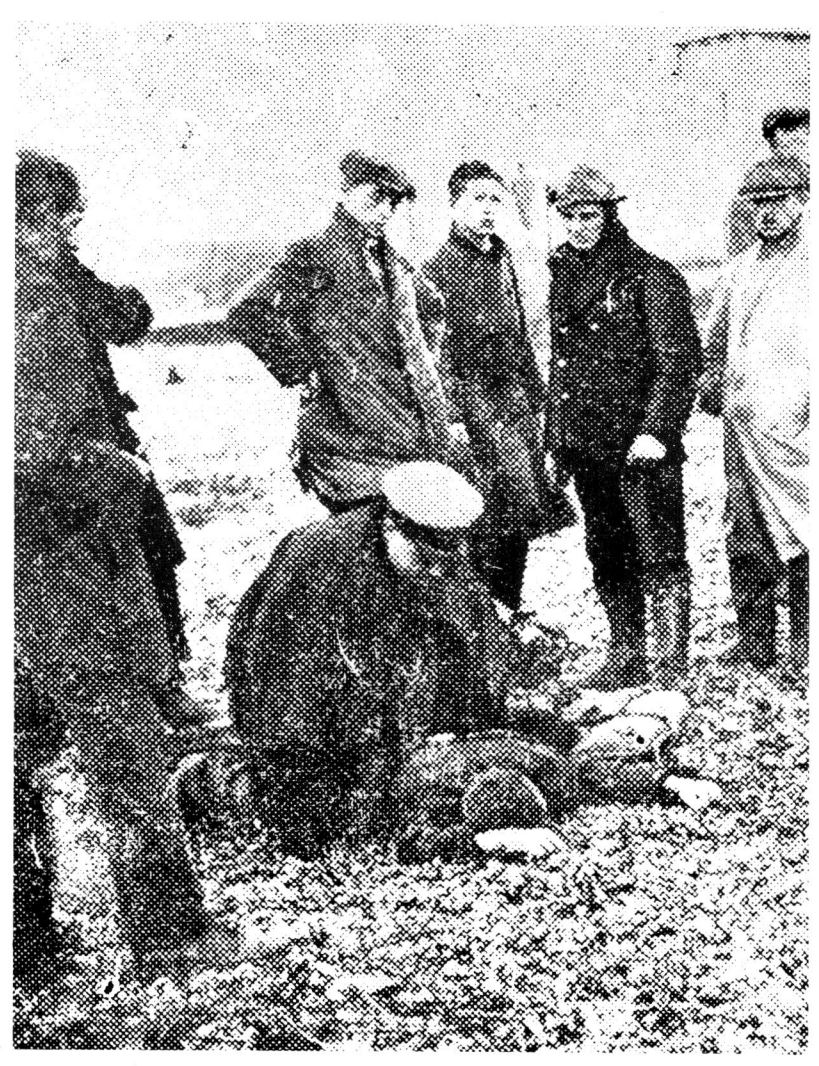

Attempts at artificial respiration were carried out on the beach

too late to save any of them. It was not so much a case that the men had drowned; they had been battered to death by the waves. Women raced to the beach for news of their loved ones and their anguished cries could be heard above the roar of the wind, waves and teeming rain. An eye-witness told of the heart-rending sight of the vicar kneeling in prayer with the women of the village.

The bodies of the lifeboatmen continued to be washed in at regular intervals during the next two hours. Helpers waded out into the water to pull them ashore. In all 15 bodies were recovered that day and after formal identification at Lydd, were eventually brought back to Rye Harbour and laid in coffins in the Fishermen's Institute.

The close-knit community of Rye Harbour that day had lost an entire generation, 11 children were left fatherless and nearly every family in the village was touched by the tragedy. The RNLI sent its deputy inspector of lifeboats to the scene and efforts were made to provide for the immediate needs of the distressed families.

King George V and The Prince of Wales sent letters of sympathy and many other messages of condolence came from all parts of the country and from foreign lifeboat societies.

And what became of *The Alice*? The empty vessel had drifted towards the shore at Dungeness where she broke up and sunk beneath the waves. Her crew — the men *The Mary Stanford* had gone to assist — were eventually put ashore, safe and well, at Antwerp in Belgium, when the storm had abated.

The upturned boat

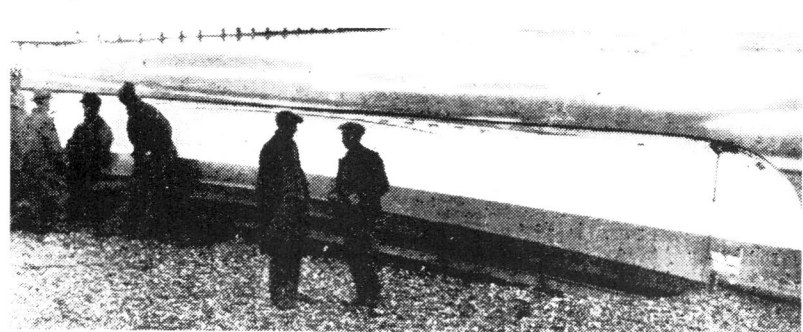

The inquest

The inquest was opened on the evening of Friday, November 16. The weather was still bad as the shocked community gathered together before the Rye Borough Coroner, Dr T T Harratt.

Searching questions were asked about the seaworthiness of *The Mary Stanford* but it was emphatically stated that the boat and her crew were absolutely efficient. After hearing formal evidence of identification, eye-witness accounts of the recall procedure and the sad tales of the desperate attempts to revive the lifeboatmen as they were washed ashore, the Coroner adjourned the inquest until the following evening.

When the proceedings resumed the main topic of discussion was the suitability of the life-jackets worn by the men. Major Hacking made serious criticisms of the lifebelts provided by the Royal National Lifeboat Institution, saying that the belts were perished, with the result they quickly became water-logged and lost their buoyancy and would have weighed a man down rather than supported him, and were more likely to choke him.

The type and pattern of life-jacket supplied to the crew were kapok type pattern No 3, tested and approved by the RNLI. This pattern was adopted by the RNLI in 1917 and the belts were delivered to the Rye Harbour station on September 25, 1917. The crew had expressed their satisfaction after trying them in a heavy gale on October 30, 1917 and later voted by a majority of 11 to six that this was the design they most preferred.

The Coroner, in recording a verdict of death by accidental drowning, suggested that Major Hacking's statement on the belts should be forwarded to the proper authorities.

In response the RNLI immediately asked the Board of Trade to hold a full inquiry into the disaster and in the time preceding this inquiry both the Board of Trade and RNLI independently tested the belts worn by the Rye Harbour lifeboatmen.

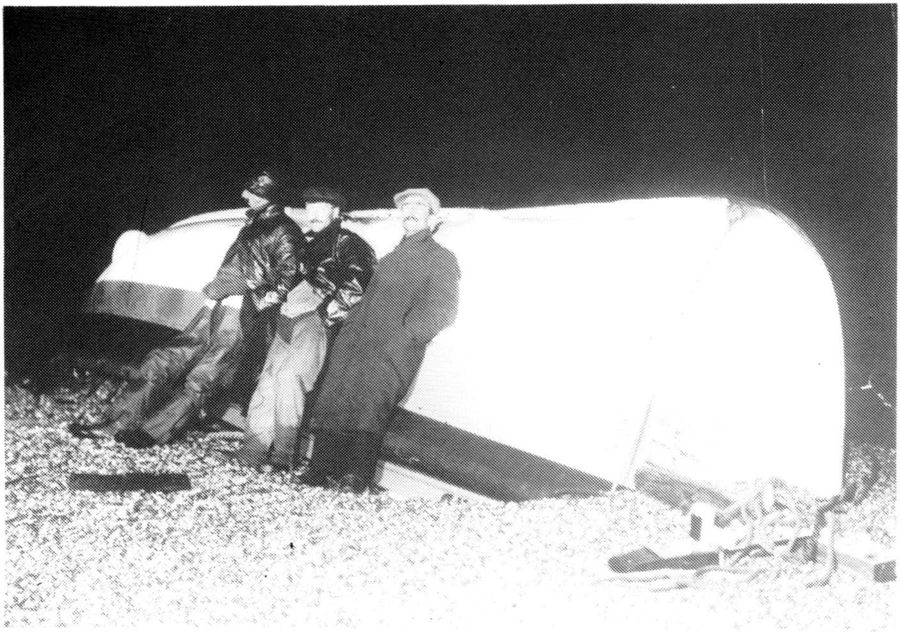

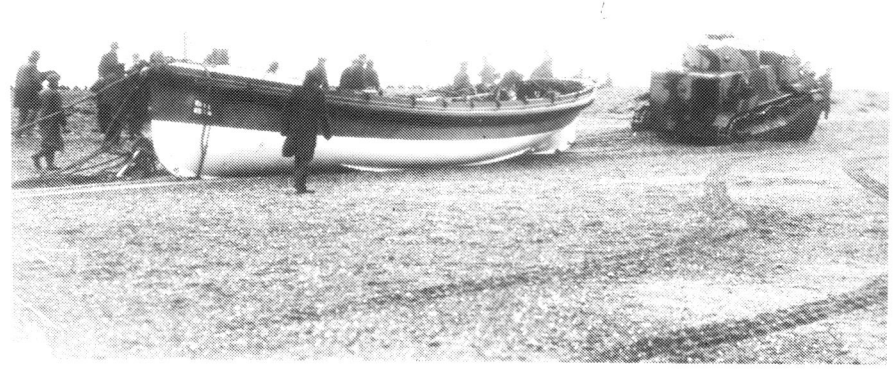

Above: The night vigil; relatives and friends waited through the following night for the sea to give up the remaining bodies. Below: The striken lifeboat is finally dragged away from the beach

The funeral

The bodies of two of the crew members, Henry Cutting and John Head had not been recovered by the time of the mass funeral on Tuesday November 20. It was not until three months later that Henry Cutting was washed ashore at Eastbourne and taken to Rye Harbour for burial. The body of John Head, the coxswain's son, was never recovered.

The weather for the funeral was fine but overcast as hundreds of people from all walks of life poured into the tiny village to pay their last respects to the lost men. Some had travelled many miles and among the vast gathering were lifeboatmen from all parts of England. It was a quite remarkable and moving occasion and the village of Rye Harbour had never seen so many people at any one time.

At 1.30pm the flag-draped coffins were brought out from the Fishermen's Institute into the street and placed on a row of iron trestles. The 120 pall bearers were drawn from other lifeboat crews, inhabitants of the village and members of the British Legion and shortly before 2 o'clock the coffins were raised to the shoulders for the short walk to the church, where the men would be laid to rest in one grave. The crew of *The Mary Stanford* had grown up together, worked and laughed together, died together and now, on this saddest of days, were to be buried together.

The Rye Town Band led the solemn procession with the strains of 'Abide With Me' and before the service began, an Imperial Airways cross-Channel airliner swept low over the village in salute.

Owing to the size of the crowd it was impossible to use the church. The whole service was taken at the graveside and divided between the Rev John Fowler, Vicar of Rye and the Rev Harry Newton, Vicar of Rye Harbour.

Members of the Latvian Government were among the dignitaries present, in recognition that the men had lost their lives going to the

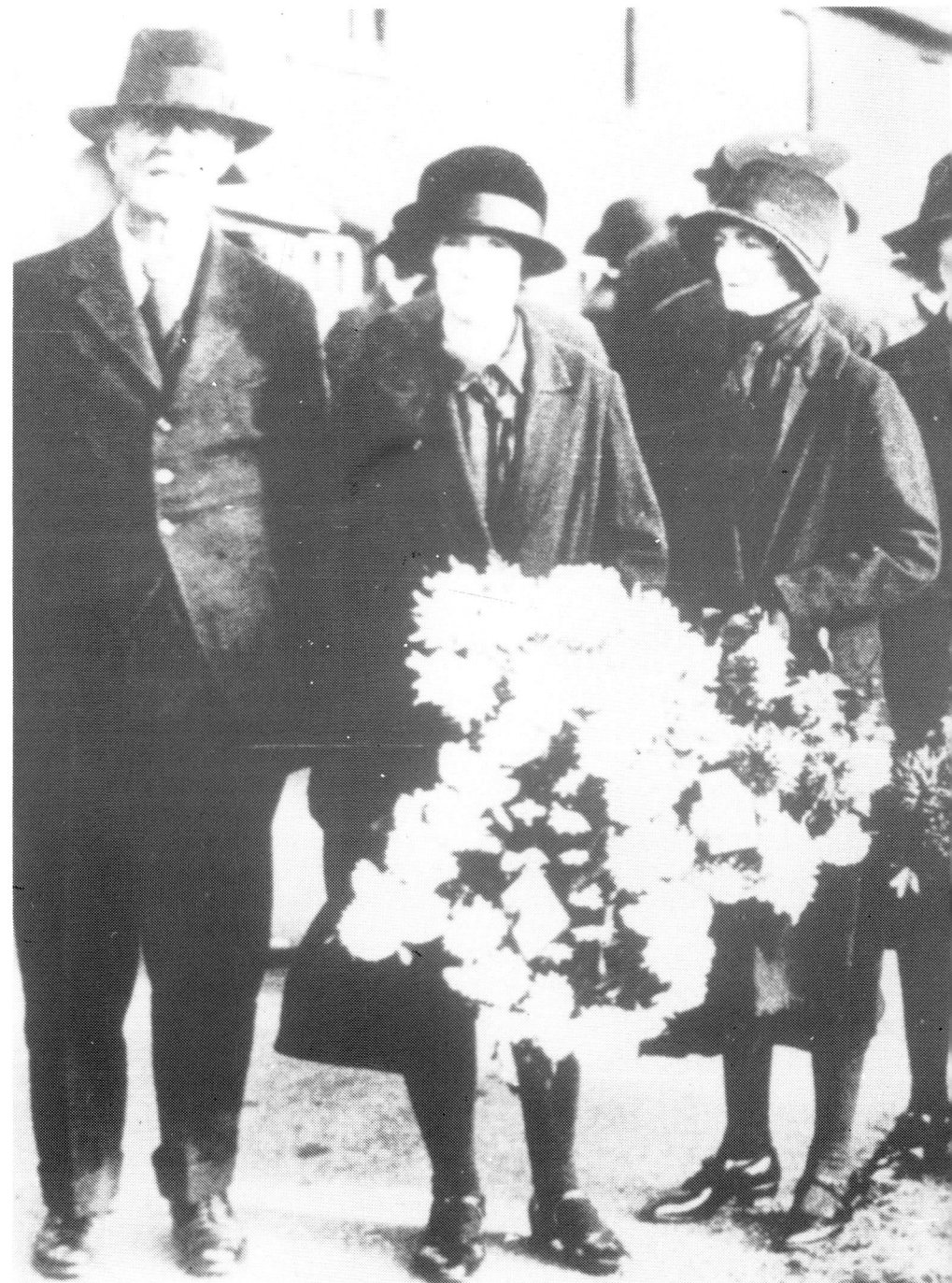

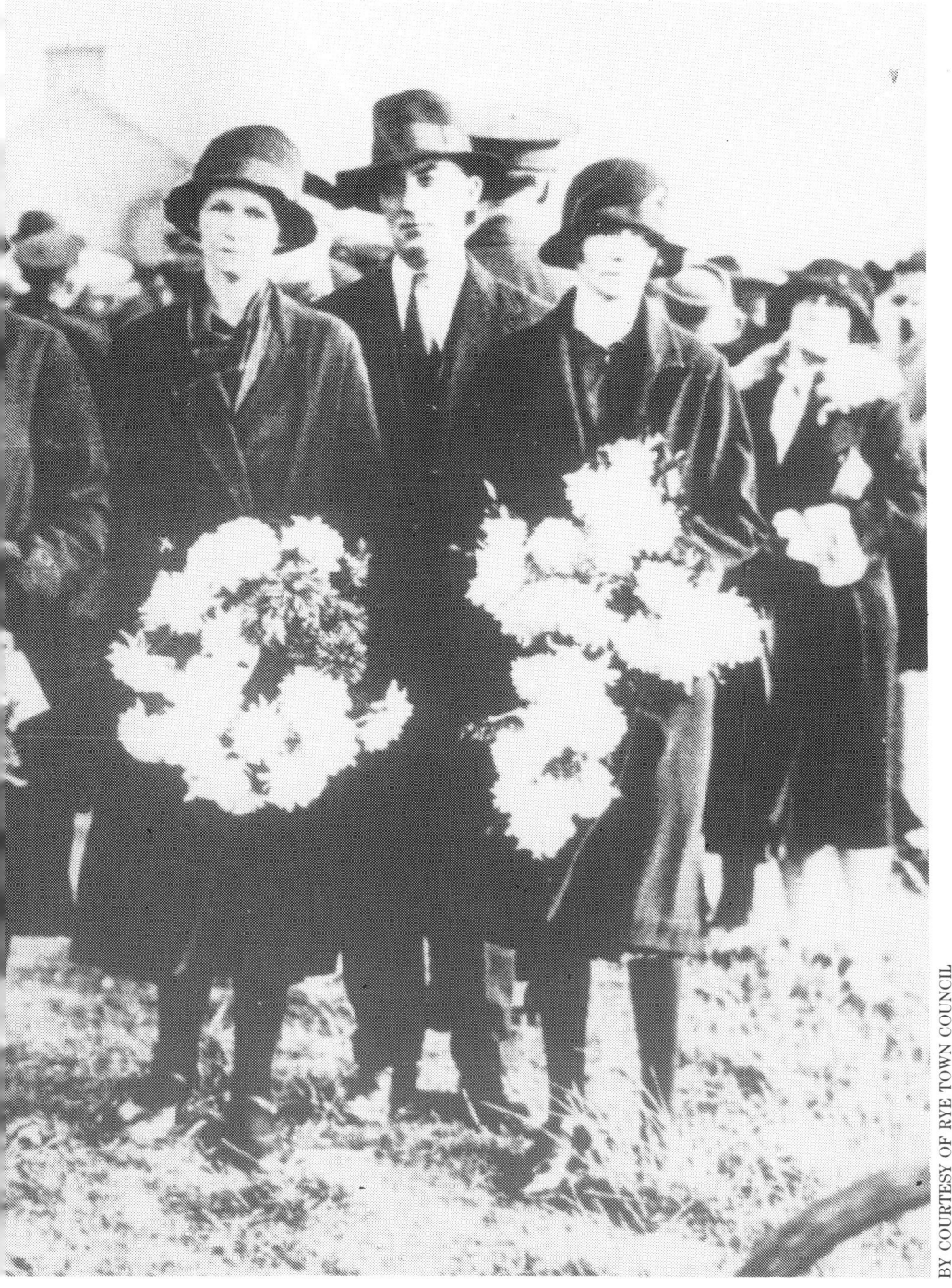

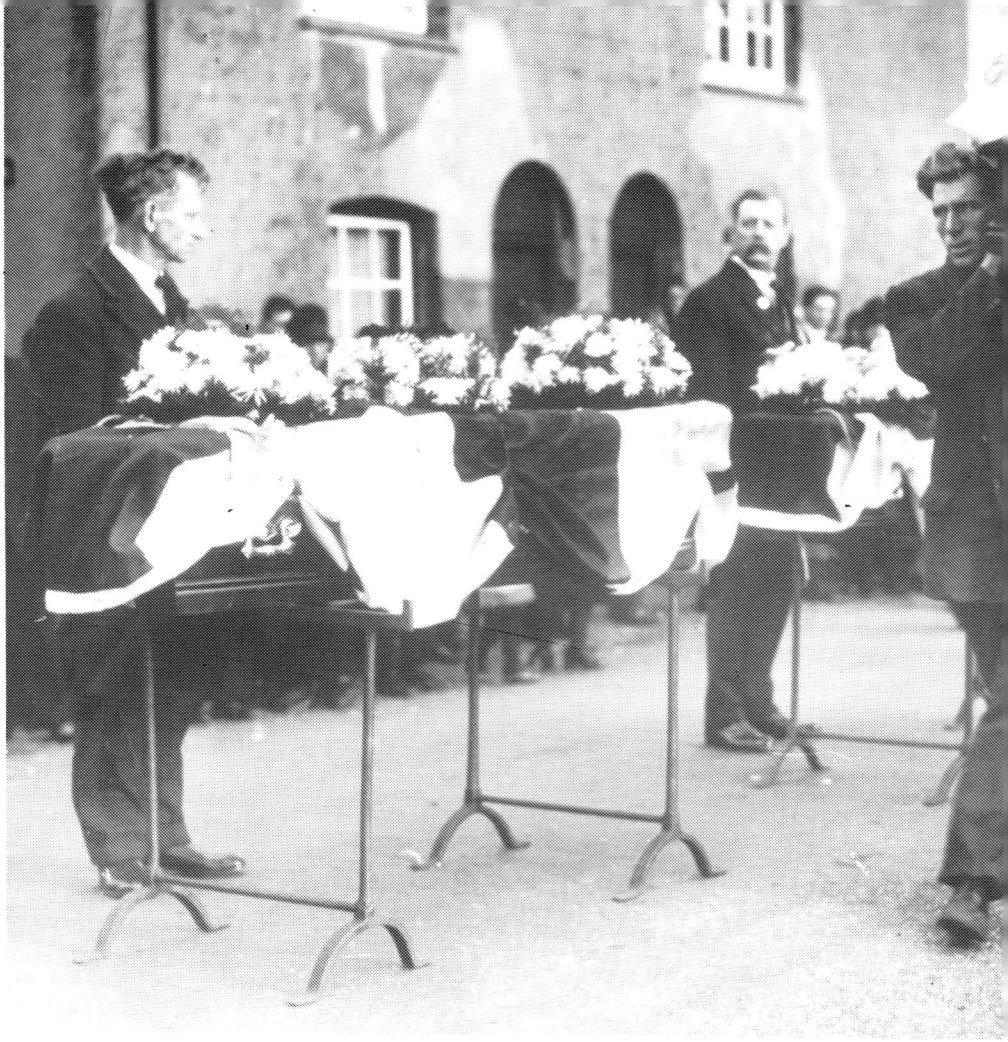

assistance of a Latvian vessel. A laurel wreath bound with national colours was laid at the graveside.

The grave had been decorated with evergreens and flowers and every available space inside and out of the tiny church was ablaze with the colour from a thousand floral tributes.

As the flags were removed from each of the coffins the simple inscription 'Died Gallantly' could be seen alongside the name of the crewman. Mrs Newton later recalled the intense emotion — and total silence — which fell over the scene as the men were lowered into the

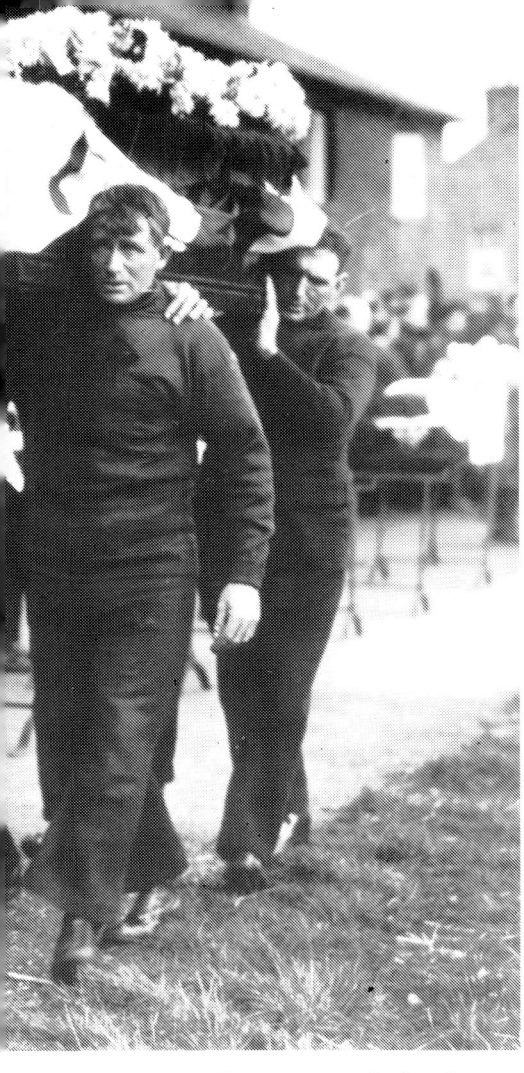

The coffins were brought from the Fishermen's Institute and placed on iron trestles in the street

grave. Tears stained the faces of hardened lifeboatmen as they quietly bade their last farewell to their former colleagues. 'You could have heard a pin drop, there wasn't a sound.'

The Rev Newton wrote in the Rye Harbour, Camber and Broomhill magazine of December 1928: 'It did not seem as if our heroes were being put into an ordinary grave. Never before have I stood by such a beautiful grave, and never before have I attended a funeral where the respect to the dead seemed so universal or more real. Everyone seemed to recognise that we were laying aside a band of brave men who had given their lives in an attempt to save the lives of others, and they were honoured for what they were. Their names will be held in honourable remembrance for many, many years to come.'

The grave now stands as a memorial to the men. A statue of a lifeboatman stands above it with the inscription: 'We have done that which was our duty to do' on the headstone. It was unveiled in 1931.

A memorial service was held on the Sunday evening of November 25 and the church was packed to its fullest capacity. A similar service is still held each year on the Sunday nearest to the anniversary.

The crew of The Mary Stanford had grown up together, worked and laughed together and now, on this saddest of days, were buried together

---

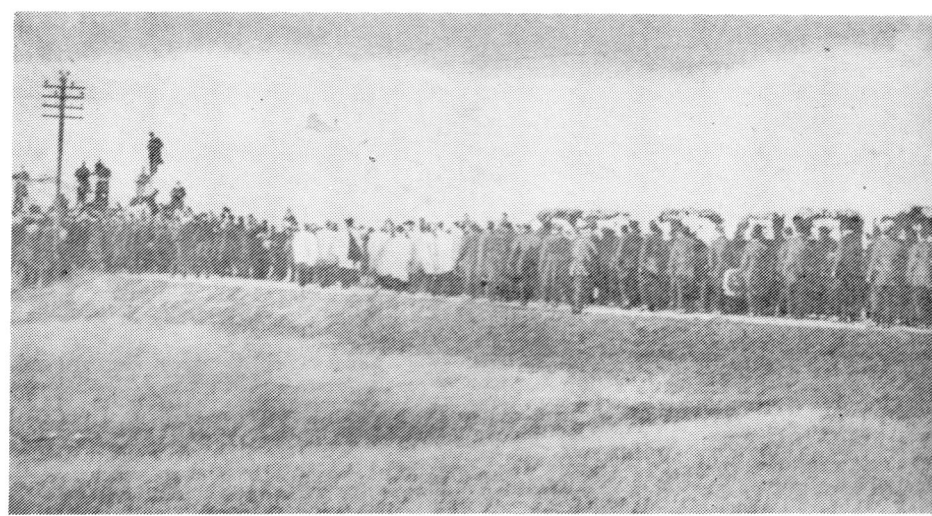

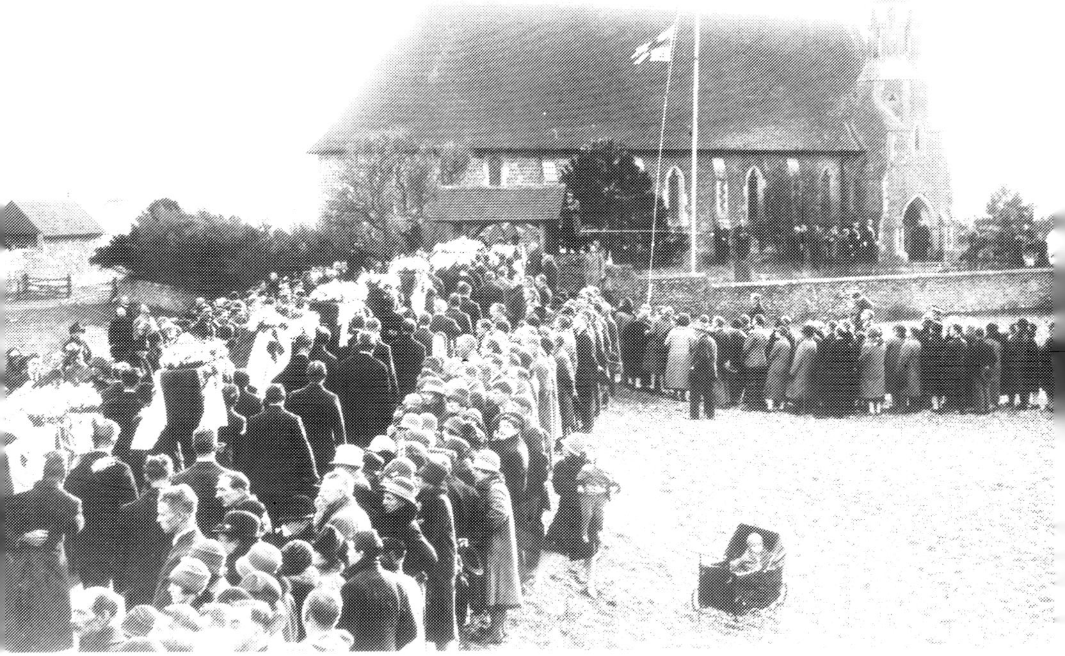

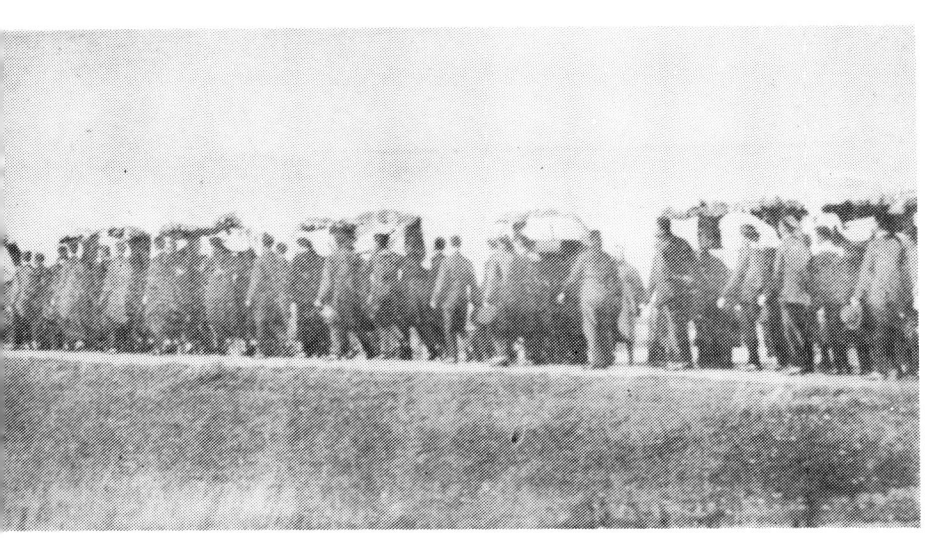

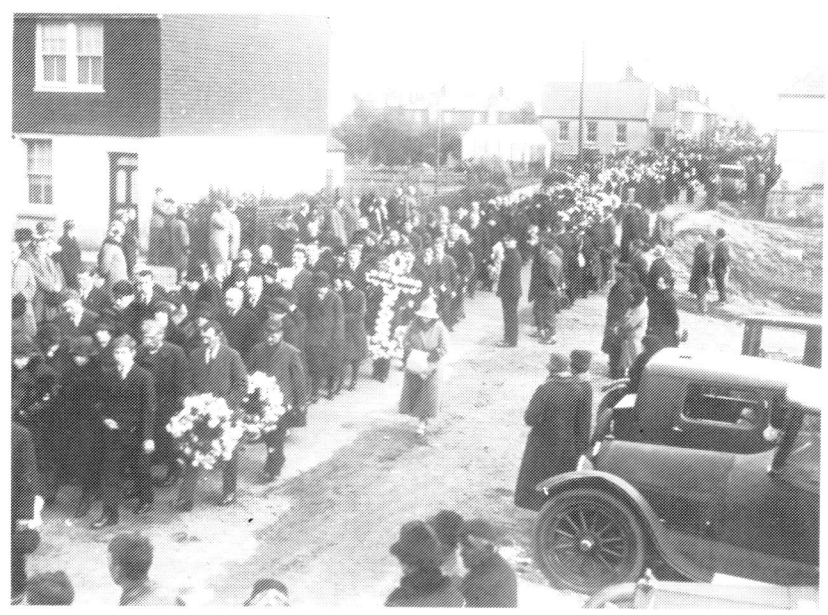

A thousand floral tributes were on view at the funeral. Above: The procession of mourners. Below: The interior of the church

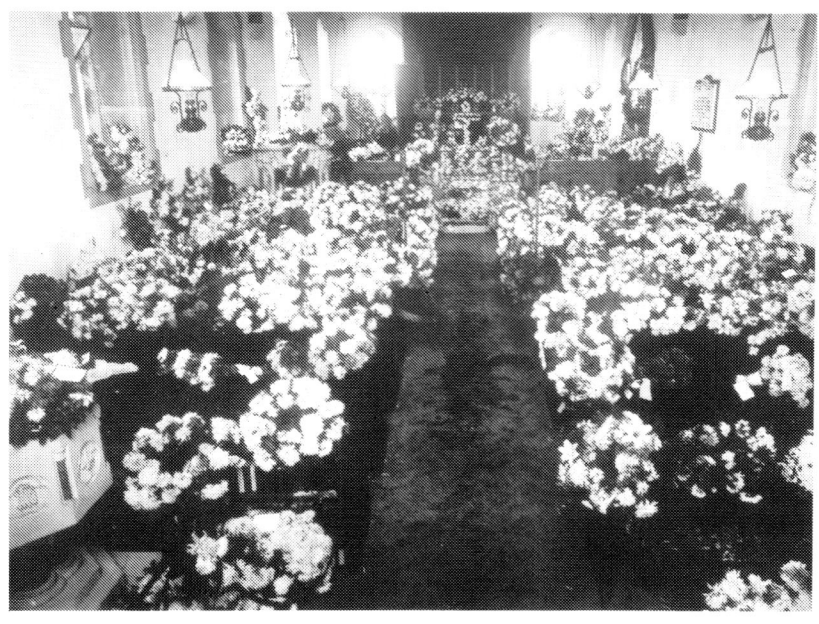

The inquiry

The Board of Trade Court of Inquiry into the disaster sat at the Town Hall, Rye, on December 19, 20 and 21, 1928 and January 1, 2 and 4, 1929. Judge Moore Cann presided as a wreck commissioner, and had the assistance of Vice-Admiral E L Booty, Captain James Garriock and Mr E F Spanner as assessors.

Dealing with the time taken for the message to reach the Rye Coastguards announcing that the crew of *The Alice* of Riga had been saved, the Court said:

'It is unfortunate that under the existing regulations it was not possible to treat the telephonic message which announced the safety of the crew of the *SS Alice* as a life-saving message. Had this been done, invaluable time would have been saved, and in all probability *The Mary Stanford* would not have been launched. Whilst we fully appreciate the great difficulty attending any extension of the class of messages entitled to priority, we would suggest that when a telephonic message involves the launching of a lifeboat the station from which the message issues should at once be informed when the crew has been called out with a view to launching the boat, and also when the boat has returned, and that during the interval any messages which may affect the lifeboat or its proceedings should be given priority as life-saving messages.'

The RNLI were naturally delighted with this change to the regulations governing this type of message, as they felt the existing rules had caused an unnecessary delay.

On the subject of recall signals the court found that the prompt and proper measures were taken to recall the lifeboat, but the recall flag should have been hoisted at daybreak, although it is highly improbable that it would have been seen.

'The recall signal was not answered by the lifeboat. Whether the signal was observed by the crew and, if so, why they did not answer, was considered to be a matter of conjecture. It was agreed that in the existing atmospheric conditions it was probably not seen.'

The inquiry considered the position of the hand-holes on the underside of the boat which would have enabled the men to cling to the upturned boat, and stated:

'With regard to the conditions which followed the overturning of the boat, it has been agreed that the men would have attempted to get hold of her. Hand-holes, in hand battens 21ft 6ins long, one on each side of the boat, were provided to enable the men to get a grip of the boat, but it would appear from the drawings that these hand-holes are some distance from the waterline of the upturned boat. In evidence it was stated that the keel of the boat would be from 2ft 3ins to 2ft 9ins above the waterline. Taking the mean as 2ft 6ins, the position of the hand-holes is such that amidships these hand-holes are about 5ft 3ins from the waterline measured along the girth of the boat. At the ends of the hand battens the measurements are about 3ft. At such distances from the waterline there is some doubt as to whether the men would find it possible to reach these hand-holes.

'In addition to the hand battens, bilge keels were fitted, which were 17ft 6ins long. Measured along the girth of the boat, the bilge keels were about 3ft 6ins above the waterline amidships, and about 1ft 6ins at the ends. The bilge keels were not fitted with hand-holes. The efforts of the men to seize and retain hold of the upturned lifeboat might have been aided if the bilge keels had been grooved or pierced to provide hand holds, or if the hand battens had been arranged further out from the middle line of the boat.'

On the particularly sensitive subject of the lifebelts the Court said:

'Although the Board of Trade and the Royal National Lifeboat Institution have carried out a very large number of tests of various types and patterns of lifebelts, none of the tests reproduced the conditions which prevailed when *The Mary Stanford* was capsized, and the lifebelts worn by the crew appear to have absorbed an extraordinarily large amount of water in the fabric, kapok, and/or pockets. It, therefore, submits for consideration whether further and more exhaustive trials and tests are not necessary, and whether kapok is the best material to use in all circumstances and under all conditions.'

Kapok is a vegetable fibre found chiefly in the East Indies, the best quality coming from Java. It looks very much like cotton, and has a very high buoyancy. The advantage over cork comes from the fact that kapok is less restricting to the wearer.

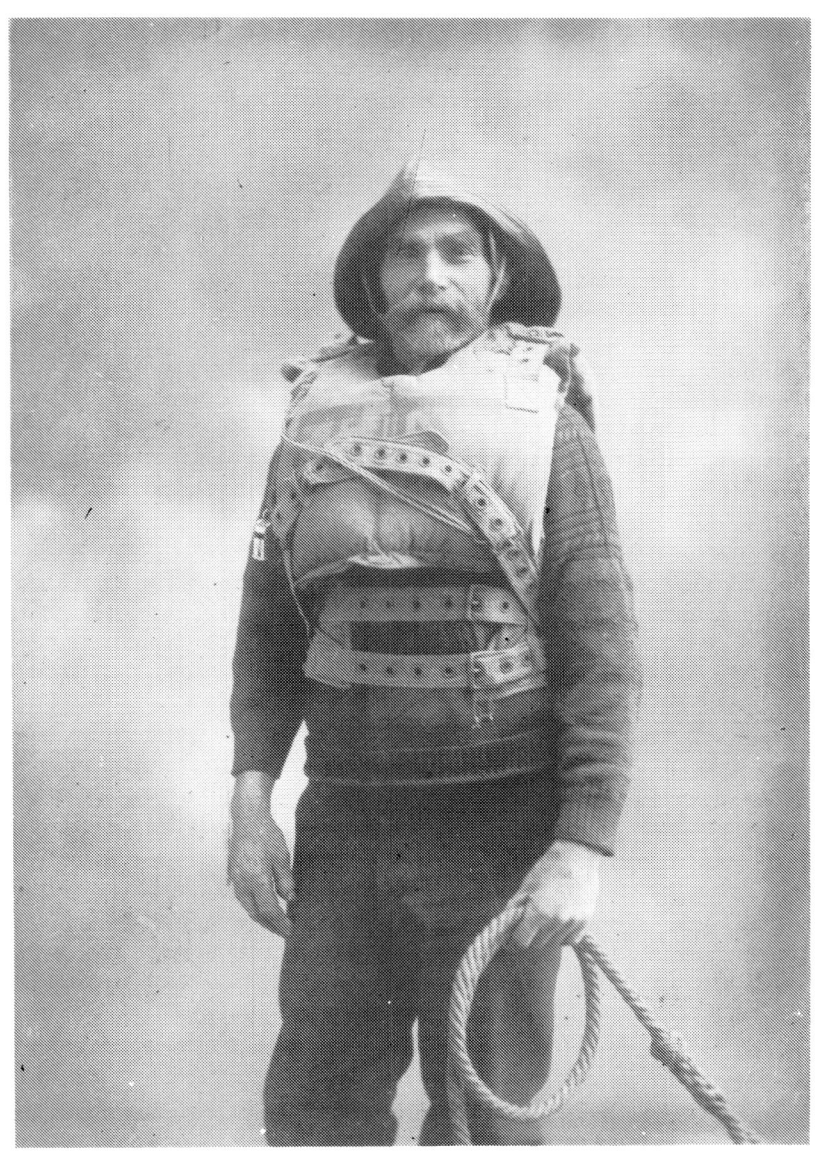

The No 3 pattern kapok lifebelt, as worn by the crew of The Mary Stanford

The Court went on:

'It being impossible to determine from the evidence before the Court how the life-jackets actually functioned after the boat capsized, the Court has made an effort to draw some useful conclusions from a study of the records of tests, etc, produced by the Board of Trade and the Royal National Lifeboat Institution.

'The Court is reasonably satisfied that at the time when floating objects, which proved to be belts containing bodies, were first sighted some distance from the shore, the particular belts around those bodies were capable of supporting, in fresh water, at least 18lb. That is to say, those belts still retained 18lb of buoyancy after having survived the battering and buffeting of heavy broken seas. Probably a further part of their buoyancy was lost when the belts and bodies came within the influence of the waves actually breaking on the shore.

'There is evidence that some of the life-belts picked up after the Rye disaster were "heavy", that they were "hard", and that they had "swelled". None of this evidence is inconsistent with the reports and extracts quoted above. It is common ground that if the buoyancy of the front pads of the belts had been impaired to a greater extent than the buoyancy of the back pads, the bodies would not have floated upright. It is common ground that if the belt pads had expanded to such extent as to press appreciably upon the chests of the men, their breathing would have been hampered. There is some ground for considering that the stability of a man when floating upright by reason of support given by a kapok belt will tend to become less or disappear altogether if the belt becomes heavy with water while still retaining its buoyancy. This point is not easily determinable by calculation.

'Without prejudging the results of such further consideration as may be given to the matter, the Court would recommend that, until there is definite evidence that kapok life-jackets, in non-watertight canvas covers, are capable of withstanding such rough treatment as may reasonably be expected to befall them in lifeboat disasters, it would be prudent to follow the advice of the National Physical Laboratory and water-proof the covers of such kapok life-jackets as are retained in the lifeboat service.

'The Court strongly recommends that, in future designs of life-jackets, the pockets containing buoyant material should be so arranged that, even if these should expand for any reason, such expansion will not result in an increase in strain on the fastenings securing the jacket to the body of the wearer.'

However, despite all this discussion, there was a general acceptance that no life-belt ever designed would have saved men in the appalling conditions which prevailed on the morning of November 15, 1928.

After all these deliberations the Court finally announced:

'As there were no survivors of the crew, the cause of the lifeboat capsizing is a matter of conjecture, but from the evidence available we are of the opinion that whilst attempting to make the harbour on a strong flood tide, and in a high and dangerous breaking sea, she was suddenly capsized and the crew were thrown into the water, two men being entangled under the boat. The broken water and heavy surf caused the loss of the crew.'

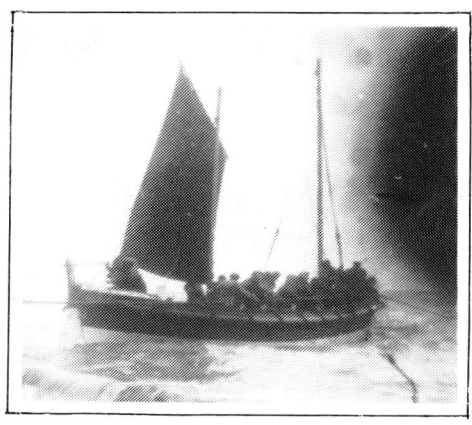

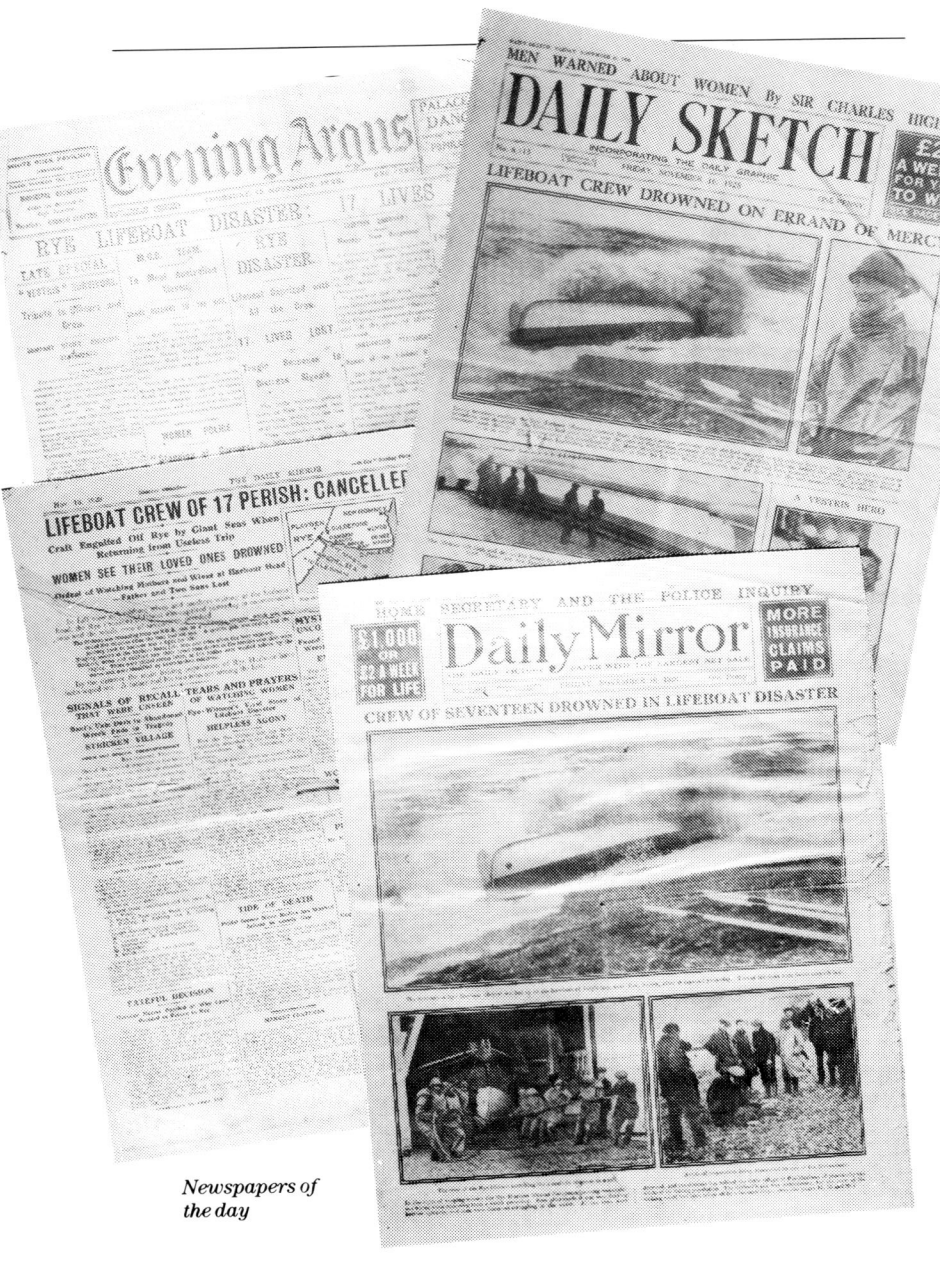

Newspapers of the day

The disaster fund

The wives, children and parents wholly dependent on the 17 men of *The Mary Stanford* lifeboat numbered 18. Each member of the crew was pensioned by the Royal National Lifeboat Institution and given the same classification as military personnel killed in action; the coxswain was classified as a Chief Petty Officer or Colour Sergeant, the second coxswain as a Petty Officer First Class or Sergeant, the bowman as Petty Officer Second Class or Corporal and the lifeboatmen as seamen or privates.

For 18 years the Mayor of Rye had held the office of local Honorary Secretary to the Royal National Lifeboat Institution, and immediately after the disaster opened a fund for the dependants. Such was the impact of the disaster, that donations poured in and the Town Hall was taken over as a receiving point for cheques, postal orders and notes. The response to the appeal was so generous that in less than a week over £20,000 had been collected. By the time the appeal was closed, some two months later, over 12,000 people had subscribed a total of £35,000.

The Vicar of Rye Harbour, who was one of the trustees, was given permission to deal with all the immediate needs of the dependants. He also took on the task of acknowledging all donations sent in, however large or small. It was a mammoth undertaking. They came from all parts of the world; one letter from Australia was simply addressed 'Rev Harry Newton, BA, England'. In order that the replies be kept on a personal level, the vicar adamantly refused to let his helpers send typewritten acknowledgements. He insisted that handwritten letters of thanks be sent to everyone who had donated to the fund; even youngsters who had sent as little as a few pence.

The Mayor, the Vicar of Rye, the Vicar of Rye Harbour, the Town Clerk and Honorary Treasurer to the local branch of the Royal National Lifeboat Institution, who were trustees, were now faced with the considerable task of distributing the money. A scheme was eventually agreed upon, and the balance of the fund was handed over to the Public Trustee, with a local advisory committee.

Reflections

There have been many shipwrecks and disasters in the dangerous waters of Rye Bay, but none before or since have ever touched a community as did the sad loss of *The Mary Stanford* and her crew. One day in November was to change the face of a village and even today the sadness lingers on.

There had been a lifeboat at Rye Harbour since 1852 but after *The Mary Stanford* disaster plans for a full-size replacement vessel were not considered. Instead the Hastings boat served the area. Operations from the Rye Harbour station were suspended immediately after the disaster and a decision was taken in July 1929 to close the station permanently. As *The Mary Stanford* had capsized on duty the boat was withdrawn from service and returned by road to a storeyard at the headquarters of the Royal National Lifeboat Institution at Poplar, in East London on Friday January 5, 1929, where she was eventually broken up in February 1930. The boathouse from which *The Mary Stanford* sailed still stands, on the lonely stretch of beach between Rye Harbour and Winchelsea Beach. It is thought to be one of the last remaining boathouses standing to have housed a pulling and sailing craft.

Today, the dangers of Rye Bay are still apparent. An inshore lifeboat was placed at Rye Harbour in 1966 and a new boathouse was opened in 1985. A glance down the modern crew lists shows us that the lifeboat tradition in Rye Harbour has carried on. Many of the family names are the same as those of 1928. The spirit of the men of *The Mary Stanford* lives on.

Interestingly, a third boat carrying the name *Mary Stanford* was brought into service after the Rye Harbour disaster, when the Stanford family expressed the wish to give the RNLI a replacement boat. The tiny fishing port of Ballycotton, on the south coast of

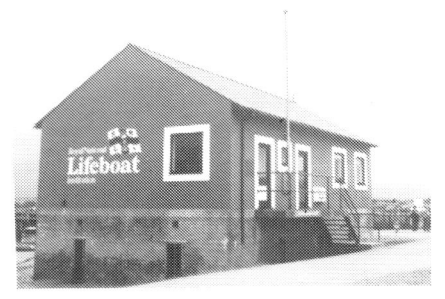

Left: The present-day lifeboat house at Rye Harbour, opened in 1985. Below: The inshore lifeboat. Bottom: Camber Sands, today a popular holiday venue and part of the area covered by the lifeboat. It was close to here that The Mary Stanford was washed ashore in 1928.

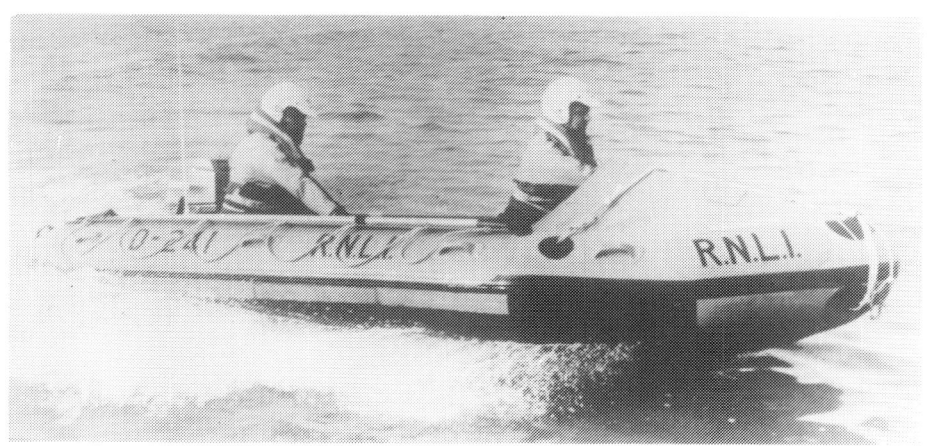

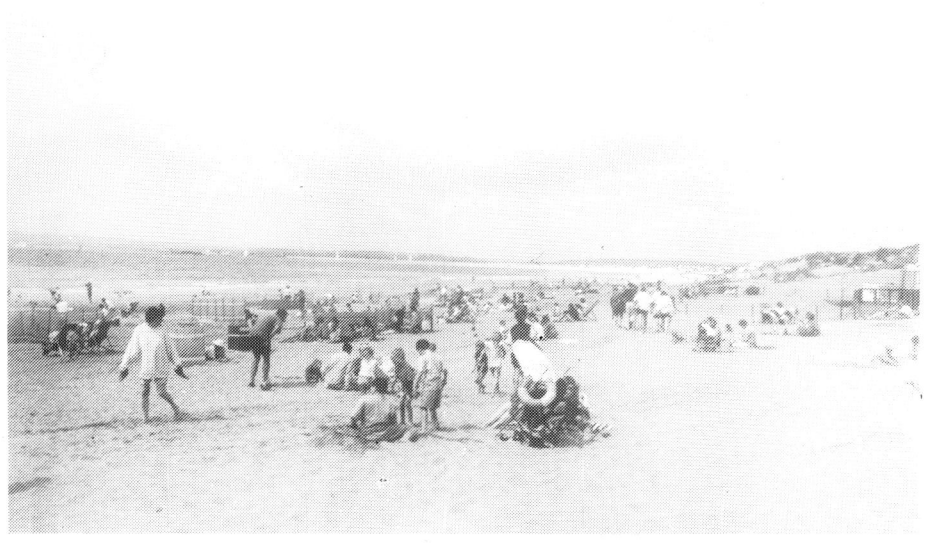

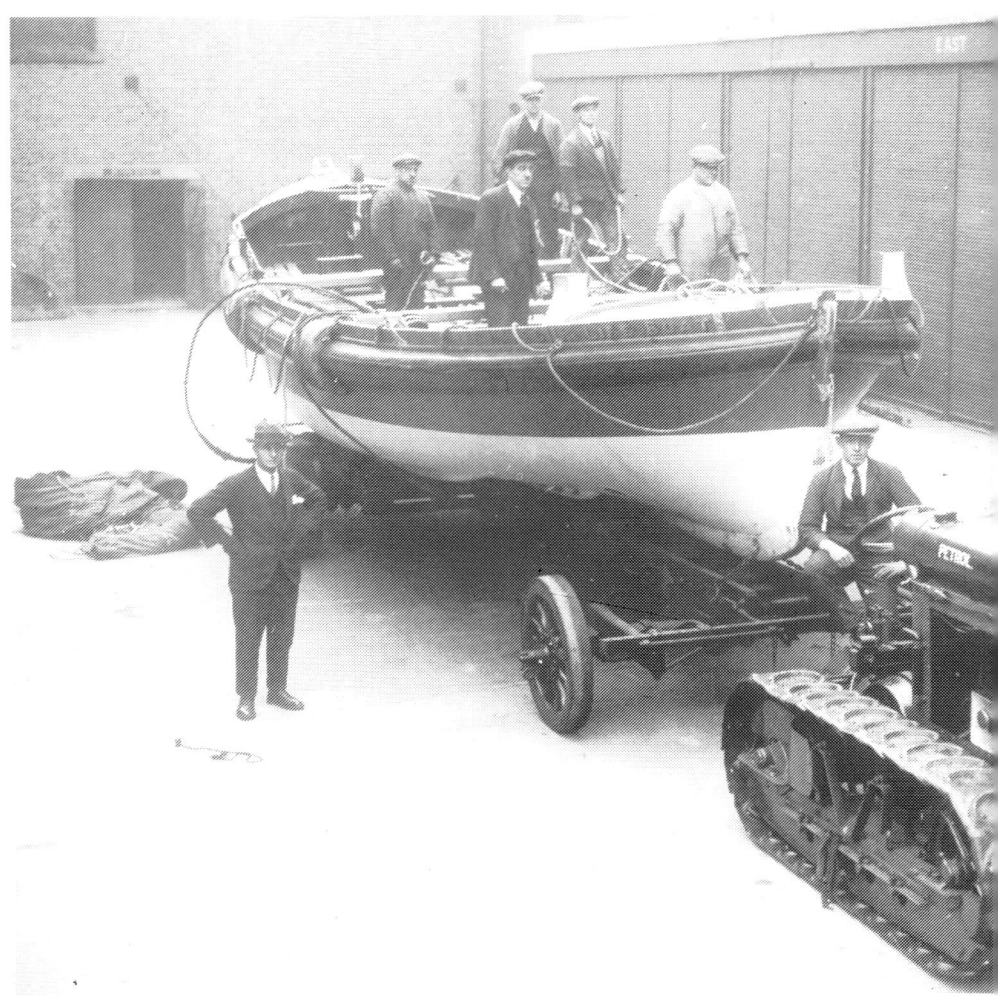

Ireland, was due a replacement boat in 1929 and RNLI officials spoke individually to each member of the crew to see if they objected to a new boat having the same name as one which had met with such terrible disaster at Rye Harbour.

The crew wholeheartedly endorsed the decision and were proud to name their boat *The Mary Stanford* as a tribute to the Rye Harbour men who had lost their lives. The third *Mary Stanford* was stationed at Ballycotton in 1930 and served for the next 30 years, during which time she was launched 83 times and saved 101 lives.

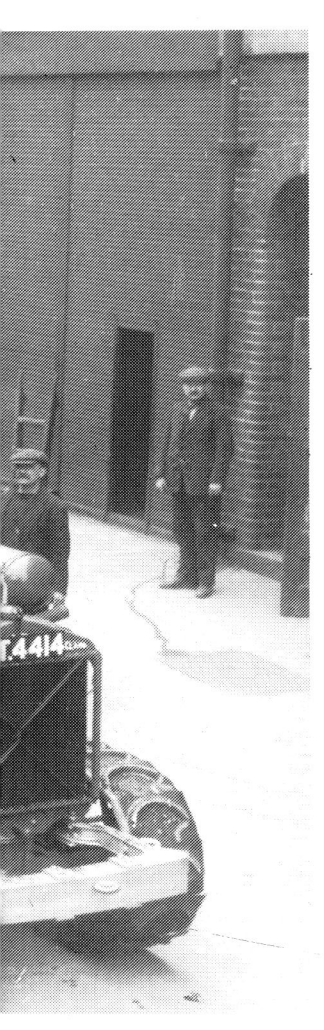

The Mary Stanford was transported by road to the RNLI storeyard at Poplar in East London, where she was eventually broken up

Apart from the memorial at the grave, there are other fine tributes to the men. In Rye Harbour Church there is a tablet of Manx stone, a gift from the people of the Isle of Man — the birthplace of the RNLI — with the inscription from the Bible which reads: 'Greater love hath no man than this, that a man lay down his life for his friend' (John XV.13).

One of the most beautiful tributes is a stained glass window, the work of Douglas Strachan, in the church of St Thomas the Apostle at Winchelsea, which was dedicated on Saturday, July 6, 1929. It

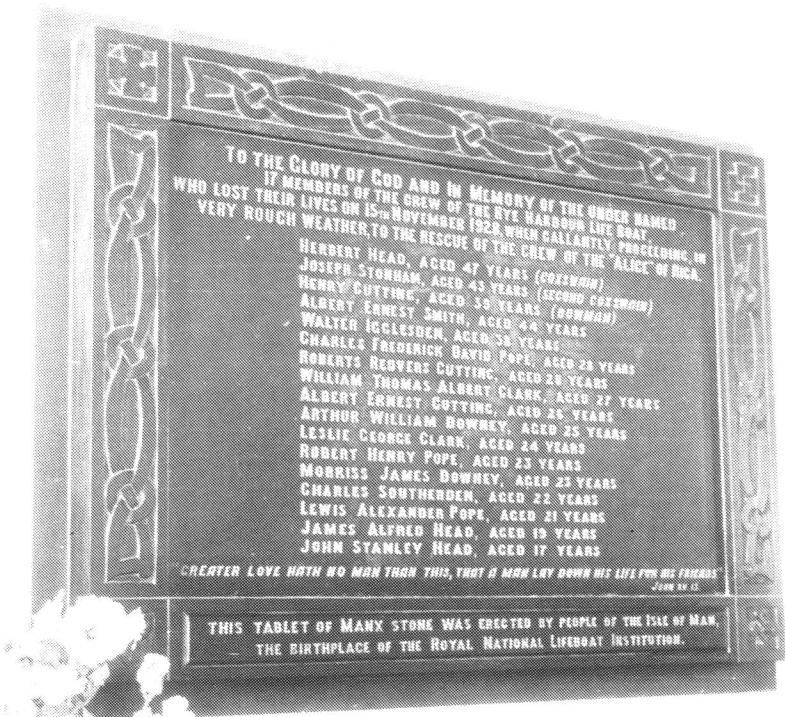

The memorial in Rye Harbour Church

commemorates the names of the members of the crew and is inscribed at the base with the beautiful composition of Sir Henry Newbolt, which provides this fitting epitaph:

15 NOVEMBER MCMXXVIII

AD MAJOREM DEI GLORIAM

These men of Rye Harbour crew of the life-boat Mary Stanford having confirmed by the habit of a noble service the courage handed down to them by their fathers were quick to hear the cry of humanity above the roaring of the sea.

In the darkness of their supreme hour they stayed not to weigh doubt or danger but freely offering their portion in this life for the ransom of men whom they had never known they went boldly into the last of all their storms.

Their names are here recorded in acknowledgement that we have received in trust for England the memory of their faithfulness and loving kindness.

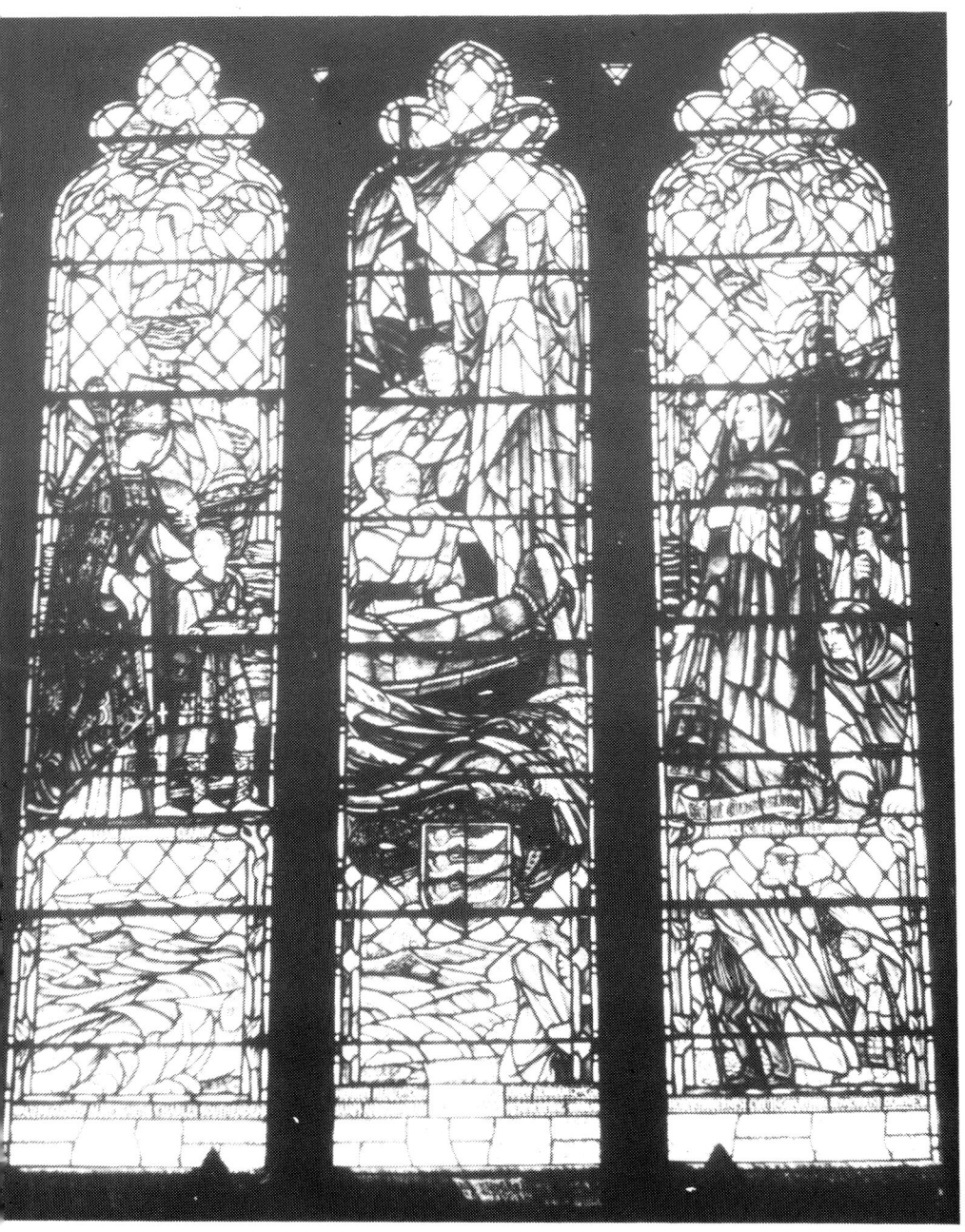

The stained glass window

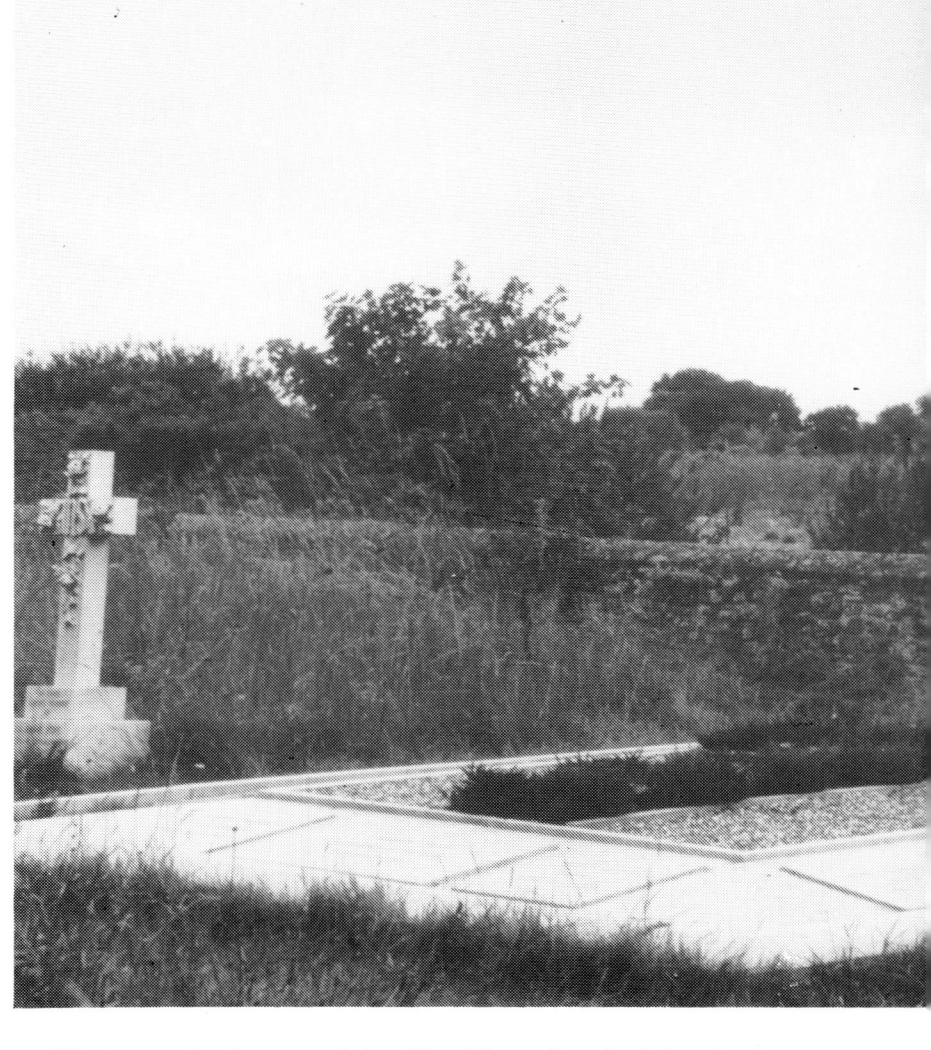

What exactly happened to *The Mary Stanford* in the hours between her being launched and her capsize we shall never really know, as none of the crew lived to tell the tale. We are, however, left with one stark and chilling fact. Had the men taken just five minutes longer to reach the boathouse the village of Rye Harbour would not

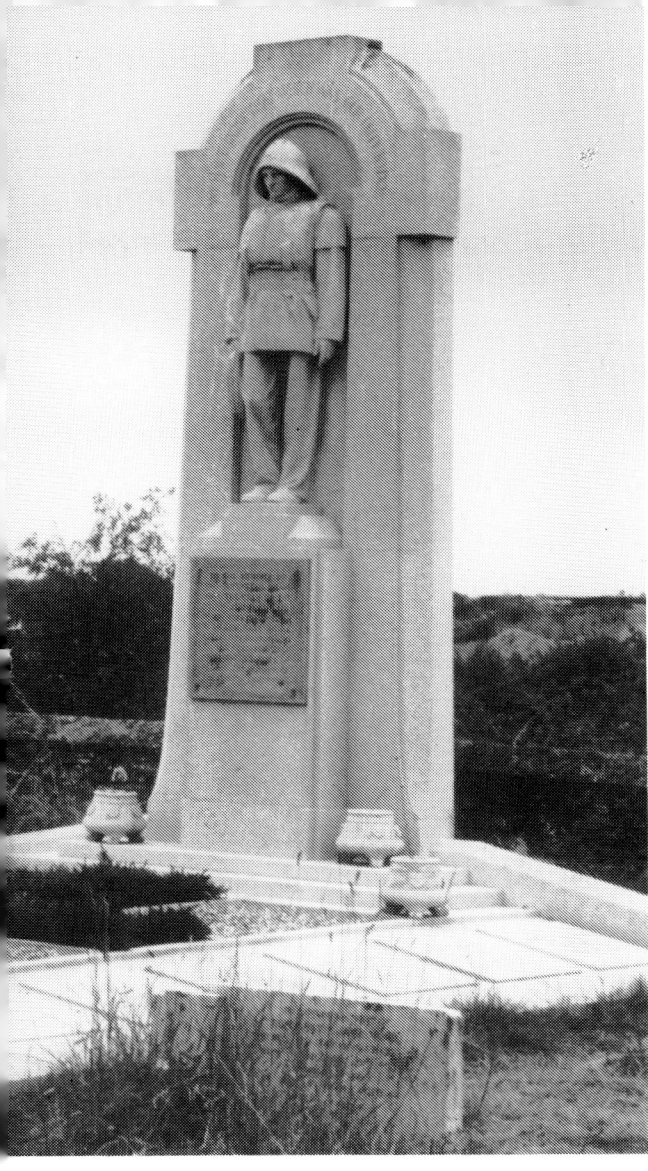

*The lifeboat memorial at
the grave in Rye Harbour
churchyard*

have suffered this tragic loss. But these were men who were betrayed by their own caring spirit; they did not know the meaning of the word hesitation and the youth of the village was snatched away in one fateful day . . .

Long may they be remembered.

Acknowledgements

I wish to acknowledge the continued assistance given to me by the Royal National Lifeboat Institution at Poole, Dorset during the preparation of this revised edition, with special thanks to Mrs Mary Gyopari. I would also like to thank the RNLI for permission to use photographs and material from their archives.

My thanks also to the Rye Town Council and Rye Tourist Information Centre; Mrs Margaret Bird and her staff at Rye Museum; Keith Fitz-Hugh for reading the text; Colin Spray and Derm Murphy of Dataset for their help in putting the booklet together; the staff of the East Sussex Records Office, Battle Library, Rye Library, Mr Ben Tart, Dave Brown, Bruce Veness and to everyone else who has offered me assistance or provided material for the booklet. Special thanks to Jan Roadnight for her enthusiasm and invaluable assistance in helping me to research the subject.

Over the years I have had the pleasure of meeting many of the inhabitants of Rye Harbour, some of whom were related to the crew of *The Mary Stanford*, and I would like to thank them for their continued co-operation.

THE LIFEBOAT SERVICE

The Royal National Lifeboat Institution is a voluntary organisation whose sole aim is the saving of life at sea. Since its foundation in 1824 many thousands of people have been saved. The lifeboat service depends for its income entirely on voluntary contributions to support a fleet of 200 boats stationed around the coast of the UK, Republic of Ireland and the Channel Islands.

Distress calls can come at any time of the year, day or night, and in all kinds of weather, putting lifeboatmen into situations which test their skill, strength and nerve as they set out to help complete strangers.

The caring spirit of the lifeboat service is perfectly summed up in the words of one modern-day lifeboatman and long-serving coxswain of the Dungeness crew, Ben Tart. Mr Tart, now retired, describes his 40 years in the service as 'a wonderful experience'. He adds — with great pride: 'No salary on earth could compensate for the feeling of putting someone's feet safely back on shore. There is no feeling quite like it.'